Bruno Pina
Paula Pissarra
Duarte Vilar

Nurses' Attitude towards Adolescent Sexuality

Bruno Pina
Paula Pissarra
Duarte Vilar

Nurses' Attitude towards Adolescent Sexuality

A Primary Health Care perspective

ScienciaScripts

Imprint

Any brand names and product names mentioned in this book are subject to trademark, brand or patent protection and are trademarks or registered trademarks of their respective holders. The use of brand names, product names, common names, trade names, product descriptions etc. even without a particular marking in this work is in no way to be construed to mean that such names may be regarded as unrestricted in respect of trademark and brand protection legislation and could thus be used by anyone.

Cover image: www.ingimage.com

This book is a translation from the original published under ISBN 978-613-9-67837-2.

Publisher:
Sciencia Scripts
is a trademark of
Dodo Books Indian Ocean Ltd. and OmniScriptum S.R.L publishing group

120 High Road, East Finchley, London, N2 9ED, United Kingdom
Str. Armeneasca 28/1, office 1, Chisinau MD-2012, Republic of Moldova, Europe
Printed at: see last page
ISBN: 978-620-8-18151-2

CONTENTS

I dedicate this work to my daughter, Benedita.

"The most indispensable thing for a man is to recognize the use he must make of his own knowledge."

Plato (n.d.)

ACKNOWLEDGMENTS

This work owes a lot to some people, for different reasons, and I would like to thank them especially:

To my advisor, Professor Paula Cristina Vale Pissarra, for her methodological guidance.

To Professor Duarte Gonçalo Rei Vilar, my co-supervisor, for being an interlocutor motivated to offer encouragement and, above all, to take new paths, listening with interest and ease to all the questions, doubts and problems that arose during the process of carrying out this work.

To all the nurses who took part in this study, without whom it would not have been possible.

To their daughter for her inspiring strength, for the love they dedicate to me every day, for being my safe haven in all my adventures, for all the strength and appreciation of my potential, for the happiness they give me, for their support, for their silent companionship in the difficult and laborious moments I've been through.

Thank you all very much.

SUMMARY

The general aim of this study was to find out what attitudes nurses working in Primary Health Care have towards adolescent sexuality. To this end, a semi-structured interview was conducted with 49 nurses working in 14 health centers in the Guarda Local Health Unit, with a minimum age of 21 and a maximum of 54, corresponding to an average age of 43.54 years (±8.33 years). The average length of service was 20.49 years (±6.512 years). *Roughly* speaking, the length of service corresponds to the length of service at the current Health Center.

The results showed that nurses have a very positive attitude towards adolescent sexuality issues. The majority said that adolescents do not approach affective or relational issues of their own volition, which, according to some interviewees, may be due to the fact that this is a subject that is usually shared with peers and not with health professionals, or because their relationships are mostly sporadic and transitory rather than effective. They also mentioned that there is a lack of maturity in matters of sexuality on the part of adolescents, regardless of gender. The overwhelming majority of nurses said that few adolescents go to the health center for sexual issues and those who do are motivated by the search for contraceptive methods and unwanted pregnancies. It emerged that the age group most likely to seek health services for sexual problems is adolescents over 15 and under 18, especially females. The majority of nurses believe that the beliefs and values conveyed by society influence adolescents' sexual freedom, as well as the sources of information, especially the internet, leading them to seek out nurses more for contraceptive reasons. They are of the opinion that there should be no age stereotype for the start of sexual life, that it should begin when the adolescent feels ready, despite the need for experimentation typical of their age. They were unanimous in their opinion that most of the time adolescents start their sex lives because of social pressure and because others have already done so at an earlier age. The overwhelming majority of nurses feel comfortable addressing issues of a sexual nature with adolescents, claiming that this approach requires adapting interventions to meet the needs of each adolescent. The majority of nurses said that promoting sexual health in adolescence contributes to the overall well-being of adolescents now and in the future.

Keywords: Attitudes; Nurses; Sexuality; Adolescents.

INTRODUCTION

The work presented here is part of the Master's Degree in Child Health and Pediatrics at the Escola Superior de Saùde da Guarda and its theme is "Nurses' attitudes towards adolescent sexuality".

Adolescence, which means "maturing into an adult", in today's thinking encompasses a combined action in which adolescents experience the demands and opportunities that affect their psychological, social and maturational development, which begins at puberty. It is, by definition, a period of development and growth, so it should be seen as a time of change and transformation and a period of life in which there are physical changes. The essence of puberty and the development of the sexual organs and reproductive capacity are experienced by adolescents as the emergence of a new role, which involves successive adaptations from a personal, family and social point of view and where there is a search for emotional relationships (Bràs, 2012; Collins and Sprinthall, 1999; Marques, 2009; Silva, 2004).

Sexuality is a relevant manifestation in adolescence, a phase of more intimate and affective discovery of the other and the creation of new emotional bonds. The awakening to sexuality is now increasingly premature. The proportion of sexually active young people has also grown. The effects of a less prepared start to an adolescent's sexual life, combined with vulnerability and risks, can have undesirable consequences, such as pregnancy and sexually transmitted infections (Bràs, 2008; Clemente, Mota and Pacheco, 2010; Sampaio, 2006).

There must therefore be a formal field of action in the development of the theme of sexuality. The school can and does play this role. On the other hand, the school, as a model of formal education and interdisciplinary knowledge, is ideal for disseminating technical and scientific knowledge that families are often unable to develop due to its informal nature, insufficient preparation and difficulties in communication between parents and adolescents (Vilar, 2005).

Sexuality can be experienced in a healthy way, but it is important that teenagers are informed and aware of all the related aspects, namely the biological ones, the consequences of sexual activity and the main protection measures, in order to avoid unnecessary risks.

Nurses have an unparalleled role to play as educators, counselors and respecters of adolescents in their experience of sexuality. It is essential to identify the importance of sex education as one of the methods that influences the maturation of the personality and the way of experiencing adolescence.

Nurses play an important role in society as one of the main health educators. The nurse's socializing role is crucial with regard to adolescents' understanding of and behaviour towards their sexuality, in order to teach them, welcome them and intervene to help them experience their sexuality in an informed, pleasurable and responsible way.

The progress that has been made in the context of sexuality in the adolescent life cycle has led to a wide-ranging discussion about what the role of nurses should be as protagonists in this development process. It was with this in mind and in the context of my work as a nurse working in the pediatrics department, with a postgraduate degree in sex education at school and in the community, that I decided to focus my study on the problem of nurses' attitudes towards adolescent sexuality, since I believe that mastering attitudes is a fundamental condition for nurses to be able to act in a way that meets the real needs of adolescents in this age group. The motto for this study stems from the fascination that adolescence has always represented and the lack of motivation and unwillingness shown by some nurses when it comes to addressing issues surrounding adolescent sexuality.

It is therefore pertinent to find answers to the concern that this raises and among which the following research question stands out: What attitude do nurses working in Primary Health Care have towards adolescent sexuality?

In view of the above, a qualitative study was carried out using semi-structured interviews. In accordance with the stated question, the study aims to achieve the following objectives:

- To know which age groups most often seek health services for sexual issues/problems;

- To find out which sexes of adolescents go to health centers the most;

- To see if the reasons why adolescents go to the health center are the same for both sexes, and if not, what the differences are;

- To know the risk situations in terms of adolescents' sexual and reproductive health that appear most frequently in adolescent care;

- To find out about the sexual content most frequently approached by adolescents;

- To find out how nurses rate their comfort/discomfort in dealing with sexual content;

- To find out what nurses think about sexual relationships between adolescents;

- To find out what nurses think about the age of sexual initiation;

- To see how sexual orientation issues (homosexual, heterosexual, bisexual, transsexual) appear in adolescent care and how nurses usually deal with them;

- To find out whether, when nurses discuss sexual issues with adolescents, they also address issues related to affections, feelings and emotional relationships, what kind of issues arise, whether they differ between boys and girls and how nurses address them;

- To see how nurses assess the level of knowledge and information that adolescents have on issues related to sexuality;

- To find out whether there are different levels of information and knowledge among young people, whether there are differences between boys and girls;

- erify how nurses classify adolescents' access to health services in the area of sexual and reproductive health;

- To know the real importance of nurses in responding to adolescents in terms of sexual and reproductive health;

\-   To see how the promotion of sexual health in adolescence can contribute (or not) to the overall well-being of adolescents now and in the future.

The study sample was made up of nurses working in Primary Health Care at the Guarda Local Health Unit.

A semi-structured interview was used to gather the data needed to meet the above objectives.

For a better understanding of this study, the body of the work consists of two parts, the Theoretical Framework and the Empirical Investigation. The first part is reserved for the theoretical background, where concepts relating to adolescence are addressed, taking into account biopsychosocial development, sexuality in sexuality, as well as nurses' attitudes towards sexuality in adolescents, using books and scientific articles and consulting *online* libraries.

The second part covers all the contents of the empirical study. The methodology presents and describes the research carried out, namely the type of study, the research design, the participants, the data collection instrument, the procedures and the data analysis. This is followed by the presentation of the results and their statistical analysis. The results obtained from the descriptive and inferential analysis are also presented and discussed. The paper concludes with the most relevant conclusions that answer the original question and objectives.

PART I - THEORETICAL FRAMEWORK

CHAPTER I - ADOLESCENTS AND SEXUALITY

1. BIOPSYCHOSOCIAL DEVELOPMENT IN ADOLESCENCE

Adolescence "is a period of transition between childhood and adulthood; it is a period of rapid physical, cognitive, social and emotional maturation, as boys prepare to become men and girls prepare to become women" (Hockenberry, Wilson & Winkelstein, 2014, p. 494).

Adolescence is a period of multiple and profound biological, cognitive, psychological and social transformations. These changes require the adolescent to fulfill certain tasks, considered to be internal and external reorganizing actions, in order to become a mature adult (Kaplan, Sadock & Grebb, 2007). These capacities vary according to different cultures, individuals and their goals. They can be listed as:

- Acceptance of body image;

- Acceptance of sexual identity;

- Developing your own value system;

- Changes in the relationship with parents - Independence;

- Development of decision-making skills;

- Development of adult identity.

Johnson (1999) divides the period of adolescence into three stages: Early, Middle and Late, as shown in Table 1.

It should be noted that the higher the adolescent's level of development, the easier it is for them to accept responsibility for themselves and others, whereas in early adolescence they have only a vague sense of *self* and are unable to relate behavior to consequences. In the middle stage he struggles with his feelings of independence *versus* dependence and often operates through trial and error, without much thought for the consequences. In the third stage, late adolescence, you can see that they already have a firm sense of their Self and can clearly incorporate abstract information into their own lives.

Table 1 - Adolescent Development

Early adolescence (from 10 to 14 years old)
1. Concrete thinking
2. Greater interest in same-sex partners, but interest in the other sex begins to emerge
3. Conflicts with parents
4. Teenagers act like children one minute and adults the next
Middle adolescence (from 15 to 16 years old)
1. Acceptance by the group is the biggest concern. It often determines self-esteem
2. Adolescents become involved in dreams, fantasies and magical thinking
3. Teenagers fight for independence from their parents
4. Adolescents behave idealistically and narcissistically
5. Shows emotional lability, frequent outbursts of anger and mood swings
6. Heterosexual relationships are important
Late adolescence (from 17 to 21 years old)

1.	The teenager begins to take a stable interest in the opposite sex
2.	Adolescents develop abstract thinking
3.	The adolescent begins to make plans for the future
4.	Adolescents seek emotional and financial independence from their parents
5.	Love is part of intimate heterosexual relationships
6.	Ability to make decisions already developed
7.	Strong sense of self, as an adult, already developed

SOURCE: Johnson (1999, p.755).

This is a stage where adolescents are presented with multiple options and where their future sexual identity unfolds. These developments take place in an environment of uncertainty and redefinition, which *roughly* translates into multiple feelings, such as anguish, fear and uncertainty. This variety and confusion of feelings is the result of the difficulty in understanding and keeping up with the physical and psychological changes they are going through (Silva & Deus, 2005).

According to Richards, Abeil and Petersen (1993, cit. by Albuquerque, 2004, p. 180), physical changes are accompanied by changes in behavior and attitudes, which consequently affect the social and emotional development of adolescents. The same authors also add that physical changes can become a source of concern, leading to alterations in the adolescent's psychological well-being. Thus, adolescents' acceptance of changes to their bodies and physical appearance can cause them difficulties and, at the same time, alter their psychological well-being (Berger, 2003).

Some studies suggest that concern about changes and the impact on psychological well-being depend on four factors: "the speed of the changes; early or late development; the ideal image; and social evaluation" (Brooks-Gunn, 1990; Caissy, 1994; Rogers, 1981, cit. by Albuquerque, 2004, p. 180).

In adolescence, physical sexual development interferes with almost all other areas, sexuality being a multidimensional phenomenon and an integral part of identity formation (Miller & Dyk, 1993, cit. by Albuquerque, 2004, p. 181).

Social development encompasses the process of learning socially responsible and adapted behaviors and attitudes, based on the rules and expectations of the various groups to which they belong. They are then able to establish and maintain more mature interpersonal relationships with peers of both sexes and achieve independence from their parents or other adults on whom they were previously dependent (Caissy, 1994, cit. by Albuquerque, 2004).

Factors such as parental practices, social and cultural expectations and certain role models disrupt social development, and relationships with peers and family are relevant (Hartup, 1989, cit. by Albuquerque, 2004). As the degree of dependence on parents decreases, the peer group becomes central to the adolescent's life.

The process by which adolescents learn to relate to others, to develop in ever larger and more complex groups, is called socialization. One of the main agents of socialization in the adolescent's life is the peer group, with whose members they explore ideas and the physical environment around them. In the group, adolescents will learn to argue, persuade, negotiate, cooperate and make concessions in order to maintain their friendships (Sprinthall & Collins, 2008).

A sense of group identity is indispensable for the development of a sense of personal identity, since adolescents have to resolve issues concerning relationships with their group of friends, even before they are able to resolve issues concerning who they are in relation to family and society (Hockenberry, Wilson & Winkelstein, 2014).

In this sense, Sprinthall and Collins (2008, p. 368) state that "the act of sharing is the basis for the emotional interdependence that adolescents usually expect from friends". In other words, the personality of friends and the ways in which they respond to each other become the central themes of friendship.

Thus, intimacy is an integral part of what teenagers see as friendship. One of the reasons why teenagers are able to achieve intimacy is because they are already able to think in an increasingly complex and mature way about others, about themselves and about the kind of relationship that can be maintained between two people.

Sprinthall and Collins (2008, p.368) state that "friendship in pre-adolescence and adolescence satisfies a basic psychological need that is common to all individuals, the need to overcome loneliness". The group of friends provides them with a homogeneous and small social group, with which they identify and, inherently, feel at ease. This integration and relationship with the peer group allows him to reaffirm his own identity, develop his social interaction skills and acquire a satisfactory maturity to integrate into society. The group also serves to satisfy three basic needs of adolescents: definition of their identity; integration into a structured social environment and emancipation from the family.

Adolescents need to feel that they belong to a group, which in a way guarantees them *status*. In other words, the feeling of belonging to a group helps them to establish the differences between themselves and their parents. So they follow the trends of the group, for example, dressing like them and wearing the same haircut, listening to the same music, among other trends.

The evidence of adolescents' conformity to the peer group and lack of conformity to the adult group gives adolescents a frame of reference in which they can display their own self-assertiveness while rejecting the identity of their parents' generation. Being different and not being accepted and being alienated from the group (Hockenberry, Wilson & Winkelstein, 2014, p. 499).

In short, the authors consulted are unanimous in stating that adolescents' relationship with their peer group allows them to learn new socialization skills, behaviours and attitudes, providing them with the conditions to develop their social skills. There is a significant identification between the adolescent and the peer group, insofar as there is a sharing of values, which are established by peers their own age, who evaluate them and do not impose certain sanctions, inherent to the adult world, from which they try to free themselves.

Adolescence, which means "maturing into an adult", in today's thinking encompasses a combined action in which adolescents experience the demands and opportunities that affect their psychological, social and maturational development, which begins at puberty. It is by definition a period of development and growth, so it should be seen as a time of change and transformation and a period of life in which there are physical changes. The essence of puberty and the development of the sexual organs and reproductive capacity are experienced by adolescents as the emergence of a new role, which involves successive adaptations from a personal, family and social point of view and where there is a search for emotional relationships (Bràs, 2012; Collins & Sprinthall, 2008).

2. SEXUALITY

The World Health Organization, referenced by Fonseca and Machado (2007, p.25), defines sexuality as

an energy that motivates us to seek love, contact, tenderness and intimacy; that is integrated into the way we feel, move, touch and are touched; it is being sensual and sexual at the same time; it influences thoughts, feelings, actions and interactions and therefore also influences our physical and mental health.

In this way, it attests to its full scope, encompassing its various organic, physiological, emotional, affective, social and cultural dimensions. Sexuality is linked to feelings and emotions, to actions and interactions, to the body and the way of being in relation to it, and influences physical and mental health. The term sexuality covers emotions, behaviors and attitudes related to the ability to procreate, social and personal patterns related to intimate physical relationships throughout an individual's life (Sprinthall & Collins, 2008).

Sexuality is seen as an integral element of each individual's identity, acquiring maturity throughout life. It is not synonymous with sex, but the result of the interaction of multiple factors, such as biological, psychological and environmental, on the individual. It has a biological function that refers to the ability to procreate, to give and receive pleasure. Self-concept, psychosexual identity and individual identity are factors that relate to the individual's internal sense of sexuality and are reflected in body image, identification with the male sex - man - or the female sex - woman, as well as learning the socially established roles for both sexes. The way in which each person experiences their sexuality is significantly influenced by the prevailing socio-cultural values and rules (Johnson, 1999). In this sense, and in accordance with Carvalho, Rodrigues and Medrado (2005, p. 378), it can be said that sexuality, as a concept, is multidimensional, referring to a psychological dimension, and is also "produced in the social, cultural and historical context in which the subject is inserted."

From the first years of life, there are manifestations of non-erotic sexuality, not in the sense of adult sexuality but of a sexual origin, which appear differently in the two sexes, linked to temperament, affectivity and personality, which evolve over time. Thus, the way adolescents view their sexuality necessarily depends on their previous experiences, the way they experience and perceive them, and above all on the information and education they receive, which they assimilate in a unique and personal way (Sprinthall & Collins, 2008).

Biologically, the human being is prepared to deal with sexuality from a very early age, but awareness of this sexuality only occurs with puberty, when functional maturation takes place. Once puberty is over, the problem for adolescents is what to do with their new body, bearing a new recognizable sex. According to Braconnier and Marcelli (2007, p.99), "...the development of gender identity is based first on the recognition and then on the acceptance of the new body image, which in itself implies content and limits". This work of recognition and progressive stabilization of the body image is aimed at the feeling of identity, which is only considered acquired when the adolescent is able to identify with the different sectors of their life.

Sexual identity is an integral part of identity and consists of the adolescent recognizing themselves in one sex. In order for adolescents to recognize themselves in their new body image and sexual identity, changes are needed in their relationship with their parents and their parental images. All of these movements condition the choice that the adolescent will make when choosing their future love partners, or in other words, the choice of sexual object (Braconnier & Marcelli, 2007).

It is in childhood that emotional affective memory is built, which will later integrate other functions; according to Fonseca (2010, p.83), ".the mother-baby relationship is the primordium of the construction of sexuality." The author considers it to be the first love relationship. The author also states that it is necessary to understand the psychological development of childhood in order to understand what happens in adolescence. With regard to sexuality, the same author identifies behaviours inherent to the different phases of adolescence, considering that the first phase of adolescence is characterized by self-eroticizing behaviour and self-experimentation; in the second phase of adolescence there is already a strong perception of the differences between bodies and a critical view of one's own body, so this is the phase in which similarities and differences are exercised, which can involve hetero, homo or bisexual experimentation. In the third stage of adolescence, emotional involvement is more unstable. In the opinion of the author Fonseca (2010, p.84), "...adolescents begin to understand, as a result of their personal experience, that through seeking out others they find pleasure, achieve intimacy and build sharing".

2.1. SEXUALITY IN ADOLESCENTS

Sexuality is a relevant manifestation in adolescence, since it is at this stage of life that sexual identity develops, where various changes take place, including physical, psychological, emotional and also socio-cultural changes. It is one of the most important stages of development in the life of a human being, where personal space is continually changing and trying to adjust. It is a phase of more intimate and affective discovery of the other and the creation of new emotional bonds. Due to the changes that take place, the contradictions and contradictions that boil up during this period, adolescence is, by its very nature, a period of potential accidents and is seen, in itself, as a source of a series of health problems (Brás, 2008; Nelas, 2011; Sampaio, 2007; Sâ, 2007).

With the approach of puberty, sexual desire becomes more specific and there are numerous stimuli that have an erotic value; this delimits the beginning of puberty and the process of adolescence. Sexual desire and attraction to erotic stimuli lead adolescents to seek sexual satisfaction through self-stimulation or contact with others.

Belief systems, social organization and one's own ability to control the pulse or find a sexual partner define, among many circumstances, an individual's sexual conduct (López & Furtes, 1999).

The effects of a less informed start to an adolescent's sex life, combined with vulnerability and risks, can have undesirable consequences, such as pregnancy and sexually transmitted infections (Bràs, 2008; Pacheco, Mota & Clemente, 2010; Sampaio, 2006).

During adolescence, the factors that have the greatest influence on the construction of sexual identity are the family and the peer group. Peers influence the adolescent's sexuality by transmitting more permissive or restrictive norms through the role models they provide. The family, especially the quality of the mother-child relationship, is an important predictor of adolescent sexual behavior, as is the absence of parents and little adult supervision (Lemur & Galamba, 1998, cit. by Canavarro & Pereira, 2001).

Paixao (2005, p. 39) states that "girls' first time happens mainly in the context of a romantic relationship and because they have felt desire for some time. Boys, on the other hand, separate the romantic relationship from the sexual relationship. Their motive is usually curiosity and imitation".

According to a study by Cuesta and Benjumea (2001) with pregnant teenagers, "ideas of romantic love serve to identify the boyfriend as the real one and guide their behavior during courtship." Adolescents are considered to have a romantic idea of love because, according to the same author (p. 24), "...this is the time when young people live and construct their identities. Sexual relations are a natural part of the course of a love relationship, because they associate sex with love".

Sexual behavior is associated with affective processes such as desire, attraction and falling in love. These so-called basic affective processes are the mediators of sexual activity. Desire is based on a purely instrumental interest in the object of satisfaction; attraction involves an explicit interest in the object; and infatuation involves an interest in the person as such (Roque, 2010).

It is in dating relationships that young people will experience sexuality. According to Matos, Simoes, Vilar et al. (2010), eroticism and sexuality are the basic elements of relationships of affection between adolescents. Adolescents perceive premarital sexual activity as regulating their relationships with their peers, even if it challenges the morals their parents have instilled in them. Sexual activity has become something of a normal part of teenage dating.

According to Bobak, Lowdermilk and Jensen (2007), the *media* has been influencing adolescents with regard to their sexuality. The authors go on to say that there are two reasons for starting sexual activity: increased sexual desire and early menarche. Girls start their sexual lives with the aim of establishing a relationship based on trust, not believing that they can become pregnant. They look for a family structure and immediately think about possible alternatives in the event of pregnancy (Bobak, Lowdermilk & Jensen, 2007). In boys, according to these authors, the start of sexual activity is mostly due to the need to belong to the group. "The boy may not want to be the virgin of the group" (Bobak, Lowdermilk & Jensen, 2007, p.758).

Sexuality is one of the ingredients of human growth and learning. It has been the subject of multiple approaches from a moral and philosophical, aesthetic, literary and artistic point of view. It's not just limited to reproduction, it's much broader, emerging in affective, social and psychic life, in sexual roles, interpersonal relationships, in distinctions and stereotypes linked to gender or sexual choice (Nelas, 2011; Vilar & Souto, 2008).

In this context, Antunes (2007) points out that, between the 1960s and 1980s, there was an increase in sexual activity among adolescents and a decrease in the age of first sexual intercourse. Adolescents began to dissociate sexuality from marriage and procreation, which led to a society that was more tolerant of young people's sexuality. According to the same author, there have been some transformations in recent years. In terms of sexuality, pleasure, experimentation and even some transgression are currently valued, in other words, all kinds of sexual behavior are approved. In this way, there is a difference between this and previous generations, with a tendency to value the erotic-hedonistic dimension of sexuality, especially among teenagers.

As the Foreword to the *Online Study of Young People's Sexuality* Report (OSYS, 2013) states, until recently, there were few studies on the sexuality of young people in Portugal, which resulted, in the vast majority of cases, in a mythologized view of young people's sexual behaviour and their, presumably deficient, preventive behaviours. According to the same bibliographic support, important studies have been produced in recent years that have confirmed what was suspected, revealing aspects of the reality of young people in these areas of life and growth. In OSYS (2013), it is clear that the majority of young people who have sex do so in an integrated way, predominantly in the context of romantic relationships, which demolishes the preconceived idea that young people's sexual relationships are mainly occasional. The same report states that only a minority of adolescents, or around 12%, report that they felt pressured to start sexual relations, suggesting that starting sexual relations is an imminently personal decision and not the result of peer group pressure. It was also confirmed that there is a significant minority of adolescents, especially girls, who have a homosexual or bisexual orientation or who declare that they have already had sexual relations with people of the same sex. Adolescents' sexual behavior appears to be coherent with their attitudes towards sexuality, most of which are characterized by a high degree of liberalism and positive acceptance of sexuality, particularly youth sexuality.

2.2. RISKS TO THE SEXUAL AND REPRODUCTIVE HEALTH OF YOUNG ADULTS

Fernandes (2005) mentions that at the beginning of the 21st century, the largest generation of young people to date emerged, around 3 billion under the age of 25, corresponding to approximately half of the world's population. The same author points out that sustainable development, with the inclusion of the social, economic and environmental dimensions, has become an issue for young people's sexual and reproductive health, and is therefore a fundamental element, given that more than 1.7 billion women worldwide are in their productive and reproductive years. These assumptions lead Fernandes (2005) to state that this is both a question of sustainable development and a question of human rights and gender equality, since the goal of eradicating extreme poverty, as set out in the Millennium Development Goals, depends on the exercise of individual rights. In this context, the author refers to the Cairo Conference (1994), where a commitment was made to make reproductive health universal by 2015 at the latest. At this conference, there was unanimity on the idea that reproductive rights should occupy a central place in human rights, sustainable development, gender equality and women's empowerment.

Fernandes (2005) also points out that reproductive health is a widely accepted term and reproductive rights have been discussed at length at various United Nations conferences. In the case of the European Union, with regard to development cooperation, it often refers to the Cairo Conference and the Beijing Platform for Action in order to make reproductive health a priority on the agenda.

Still in this vein, Fernandes (2005) refers to the need to further promote psychosocial health and reproductive health needs, which implies avoiding exposing girls to physical and sexual abuse, combating gender-based violence and female genital mutilation, minimizing emotional pressures regarding sexuality, among others. She also adds that the key to healthy sexuality in adulthood also lies in the provision of age-appropriate information, which should be given progressively, so that adolescents' sexual maturation is not forced (Fernandes, 2005).

Sexually Transmitted Diseases or Sexually Transmitted Infections are another preventable problem that causes anguish among adolescents. In 2002, the World Health Organization (cited by Bràs, 2012, p.16) stated that:

In addition to violence, drug use and accidents, the spread of the Human Immunodeficiency Virus (HIV) and other sexually transmitted diseases are the biggest threat to young people's lives in the coming years. The same organization warns that there is enormous ignorance among young people about sex and the risks associated with it. We're not just talking about Acquired Immune Deficiency Syndrome (AIDS), but other diseases which, while not fatal or incurable, such as Syphilis, Gonorrhea, Herpes and Chlamydial infections, cause organ damage. Most of these diseases are not serious if they are treated early and properly, otherwise they carry risks related to the development of certain types of carcinoma, sterility and in the most serious cases can lead to death.

In 2008, Reis and Matos (cit. by Alves, 2010, p. 5) indicated that:

The increase in STIs, particularly HIV/AIDS, combined with other risks linked to sexual activity, such as unwanted pregnancy, has led to sexuality being considered a matter of epidemiological social urgency and a factor that can have a significant negative impact on health. These problems are often based on a great deal of illiteracy on basic issues related to sexuality and reproductive life.

It is essential to recognize the importance of sex education as one of the processes that influences personality maturation and the way adolescents experience adolescence.

Sexual education should start as early as possible, be ongoing and be linked to the education of all children and adolescents. It should be informally initiated and taken up by parents, complemented by schools and health professionals. It is essential that nurses address sexuality in its entirety, whether during individual consultations with adolescents, in groups or in partnership activities with the community and schools.

Adolescence is the time when sexual identity is consolidated. The sharing and receiving of sexual information by adolescents allows them to permanently construct their sexual identity. In this context, it is important to highlight the importance of anticipatory care as a health promotion and disease prevention factor (Direçao-Geral da Saù, 2013).

2.3. STUDIES ON ADOLESCENT SEXUALITY

Adolescent health is a debate that is increasingly exciting the scientific and medical community worldwide, specifically sexual and reproductive health issues. Many of the dilemmas inherent in sexual and reproductive health are linked to the premature initiation of sexual activity. However, adequate information about sexuality can help adolescents to make more cautious choices about their sexual behavior (Oliveira, 2011).

Discussing sexuality is important, but the information gathered can have positive or negative consequences, depending on the information that is transmitted, i.e. whether it is valid and appropriate, or whether you don't know how to convey the message in the best way or if you set bad examples, which can lead to risky behavior. The socialization of individuals in the area of sexuality is therefore a process in which all the actors who shape our identity in all the other areas of our lives intervene, whether or not they take part (Vilar and Ferreira, 2009; Matos, 2010; Oliveira, 2011).

Vilar and Ferreira (2011), based on their study of Portuguese adolescents, found that 42% of the adolescents surveyed said they had already experienced sexual relations in the context of romantic relationships or occasional relationships. Most of these teenagers said that they had taken preventive measures with regard to unwanted pregnancies and STIs, so it seems that preventive thinking is already part of young people's sexual experience. There is, however, a significant proportion, albeit a minority, who engage in risky behavior. There is little recourse to health professionals and services, partly because they have never felt the need. But on the other hand, according to the same authors, it could be related to a lack of information and difficulties of access. The study suggests that sexual education does not anticipate the start of sexual relations and is even a factor in some postponement. In this sense, Vilar and Ferreira (2011) state that better sex education reduces some negative aspects of the experience of sexual relations, providing a more rewarding experience. As such, they concluded that sexual education also tends to be positively associated with some preventive behaviors and with adolescents' ability to ask for help when necessary.

In a study carried out by Garcia (2011) on a sample of 3,278 teenagers from Lisbon, with an average age of 18-19, it was concluded that the vast majority (83.3%) are sexually active and that 79.2% had their first sexual intercourse at the age of 16 or over. According to the same study, boys and girls feel more comfortable buying contraceptives and bringing them with them. The pill and condoms are the most commonly used methods (70.4% and 69% respectively). More adolescent males consider that bringing condoms with them means they are planning to have sex and are less likely to refuse unprotected sex. The same study also concludes that sex education in schools is fundamental to curbing risky behavior and that classes on this subject have been fulfilling their role, as students who have had sex education classes show safer sexual behavior.

Reis, Matos and Diniz (2010) carried out a study with a sample from the national HBSC/SSREU study, aged between 18 and 35, the results of which revealed that the majority had already had sexual intercourse, had their first sexual intercourse at the age of 16 or over, and used condoms as their first contraception. The contraceptive methods usually chosen by these young people are condoms and the pill in order to prevent sexually transmitted infections and unwanted pregnancies. Boys had their first sexual intercourse earlier than girls and more often did not use any contraceptive method, suggesting a high risk of contracting an unwanted pregnancy or an STI. Men and older young people more often reported having sex with another person during their romantic relationship, occasional sexual partners, more than 3 occasional sexual partners in the last year and sexual relations under the influence of alcohol or drugs. The results reflect the need to implement educational policies in the field of sexuality, with a view to guiding young people towards healthy sexual practices. As such, Reis, Matos and Diniz (2010) stress the need to make adolescents more responsible and more attentive to caring for their sexual health, as well as that of their partners.

In this context, reference should be made to the pilot project of the Figueira da Foz health center and two schools in the municipality which, in partnership, aimed to create a space for debate and information for students on sexuality (Soares, Santos & Gonçalves, 2011). This project complies with Law No. 60/2009 and is regulated by Ministerial Order No. 196-A/2010. The creation of this support space for students was considered a priority strategy, as a very significant percentage of students were found to have misinformation about sexuality. This conclusion was reached after a questionnaire was administered to 9th grade students to assess their knowledge of contraceptive methods, sexually transmitted infections and sexuality. It was concluded that only 15% of the students gave correct answers, indicating that the vast majority of them have a lack of knowledge about contraceptive methods, sexually transmitted infections and sexuality (Soares, Santos & Gonçalves, 2011).

A study carried out by Soares, Santos and Gonçalves (2011) revealed a lack of preparation on the part of young people when it comes to sexual involvement, a feeling of invulnerability, difficulty in making decisions, low self-esteem, a lack of definition of identity and a need for affirmation within the peer group.

When confronted with a lot of information, not always explicit and sometimes contradictory, many adolescents find it difficult to interpret it and in most cases they don't have anyone they can trust to explain it to them properly. In this sense, health professionals can take on the role of sexuality educators, helping adolescents to obtain scientific knowledge appropriate to their level of development and equipping them with the knowledge that will allow them to choose healthy behaviors when experiencing their sexuality (Soares, Santos & Gonçalves, 2011).

It is therefore important for the health professional to possess certain attributes, namely genuine concern for the physical and psychological well-being of adolescents, mastery of communication skills, ease of relating, respect for the values and beliefs of adolescents, family and the surrounding community and the ability to recognize situations that require the intervention of other professionals (Soares, Santos & Gonçalves, 2011).

In a study carried out by Brancal (2007, cited by Oliveira et al., 2014), the reasons given by adolescents for having sex ranged from "to confirm love", which reinforces the importance of emotional relationships, to "physical attraction". The reasons given for not having sex ranged from "it wasn't convenient" to "for fear of catching diseases", indicating some concern about health.

In the study by Borges, Latorre & Schor (2007, cit. by Oliveira et al., 2014), carried out with a sample of 406 adolescents aged between 15 and 19, it was observed that kissing and dating proved to be almost universal in the sample studied, presumably because they tend to occur in the early years of adolescence, i.e. before the period between 15 and 19 years of age. This indicates that the first manifestations of affection, love and, presumably, the first pre-sexual experiences, which are usually present in dating relationships, happen mostly before the age of 15. The same authors refer to various studies on the subject, in particular the studies by Askun & Ataca (2007), and assure that young people allude to a series of reasons for starting physical intimacy. Girls most often mention reasons such as love and affection, while boys most often mention physical pleasure as the main reason for starting sexual activity.

In this context, Oliveira et al. (2014), through a study, identified sociodemographic variables that influence adolescents' motivation to have or not have sex, in a sample made up of 545 adolescents (262 boys and 283 girls), with an average age of 13.95 years), attending the 3rd cycle of basic education in four school groups, three in the municipality of Fundão and one in the municipality of Tabuaço. The study showed that there were statistical differences between gender and adolescents' motivation for having or not having sex. Boys are more motivated to have sex for reasons of hedonism and health, and not to have sex because of fear, conservatism/disinterest and because it is immoral. Girls' motivation is related to relational interdependence.

Similarly, schooling is significantly associated with adolescents' sexual motivation (Oliveira et al., 2014). The same authors state that the results show that both gender and schooling influence adolescents' motivation to have or not have sex. Thus, there is a need to identify the causes that motivate adolescents' choices in this area, allowing the various educational agents, parents, teachers and health professionals to develop intervention strategies aimed at the real needs of students.

An exploratory study of 680 adolescents, carried out by Ferreira & Torgal (2011), showed that the majority of respondents have not yet started sexual activity; boys are the ones who most often report having already had sexual relations; condoms are not a method used by all adolescents in their sexual relations and the majority of adolescents do not undergo sexual health surveillance. The authors also point out that it is important for sexually active adolescents to receive health care and counseling. This means that health institutions and their professionals must be proactive in order to prevent adolescents from engaging in risky behaviors that could compromise their development and their current and future health, as well as jeopardizing their entire lives. Some behaviors, which result in maternity/paternity in particular, have irreversible consequences (Ferreira & Torgal, 2011).

Although trends in the sexual behavior of sexually active adolescents have been more positive in recent years, because the use of contraceptive methods has increased, contraception is not always considered a priority issue by adolescents at the beginning of their sexual lives and there are still many who do not use them or do so inconsistently or incorrectly (Parkes, Wight, Henderson & Hart, 2007).

Adolescents may have received information/training about contraceptive methods and the importance of practicing safe sex, but this doesn't always mean that they use it. Some teenagers say they should use condoms, but when the time comes they forget. The lack of ability to negotiate abstinence or condom use and to talk to their partner about sex, the perception that the risk is low and the circumstances in which the encounter occurs (unexpected, unavailability of condoms) can lead to them engaging in unprotected sex. Condoms were the most commonly used form of contraception during first sexual intercourse. However, they found that a worrying minority of participants did not use any contraceptive method during their first sexual intercourse, which is considered risky sexual behavior and, consequently, a threat to the physical and social health of adolescents. In turn, adolescents who had their first sexual intercourse at an earlier age were the ones who most often reported not having used a condom. As the age at which sexual activity begins increases, the percentage of adolescents who use contraceptives increases (Ferreira & Torgal, 2011). In this way, these data corroborate other studies which point to the fact that early initiation of sexual activity is more associated with poor sexual education, less knowledge of physiology or the biological aspects of sex or reproduction, and is related to unprotected sex in the first relationship (Gómez, Sol, Cortés & Mira, 2007).

The aforementioned study also found that of the adolescents who said they were sexually active, the frequency of intercourse ranged from less than once a month to six times a week, with girls reporting more sexual intercourse. The majority of sexually active teenagers said they used contraceptive methods, with condoms being the most commonly used, while a smaller percentage of those surveyed used both condoms and the pill. Given the risk of sexually transmitted infections, it was found that a worrying percentage of adolescents did not use condoms in their sexual relations. The number of sexual partners ranged from 1 to 9, with the majority of adolescents reporting having only had one. Boys had more partners, while the majority of girls said they had only had one and none had had more than three. However, there were no differences in the number of partners according to age (Ferreira & Torgal, 2011). The authors concluded that there were no differences between genders, nor between year of schooling and contraceptive use. Comparing these results with those of other authors (Matos, Simoes, Vilar et al., 2010; Vesely, Wyatt, Oman, Aspy, Kegler, Rodine et al., 2004) who questioned adolescents about the use of contraceptive methods during their last sexual intercourse, it can be seen that they are in line in that the majority of adolescents use contraceptive methods and condoms continue to be the most used method.

CHAPTER II - NURSES' ATTITUDES TOWARDS ADOLESCENTS' SEXUALITY

1. NURSES AND THE SEXUALITY OF ADOLESCENTS

Nurses have an important role to play in mediating multidisciplinary actions focused on adolescent sexuality. Until recently, the only standard of sexual health was that proposed by ethics. Appropriate sexual behavior was considered to be that which coincided with the dominant moral indications, and those that were contrary to morality were considered to be maladjusted, pathological or unhealthy. Professionals simply took the moralists' standards as their own (López & Fuertes, 1999).

Nurses can act and develop health education actions, in a dynamic and continuous process, to collaborate with this age group in order to reduce unnecessary risks to their health, but in order to do so, they must be prepared to deal with this topic and the themes relating to human sexuality and adolescence.

Working with adolescents and their sexuality is an integral part of the activities that permeate the actions and behaviors of primary health care nurses, as a major requirement for carrying out their professional role. These nurses set out to work with groups of adolescents in health centers, schools or community centers, and they know that the issue that emerges with particular significance in the discussions is sexuality (Bràs, Anes, Brâs & Praça, 2010). The same authors, based on their research with 1,735 nurses working in 226 health centers in the 18 health sub-regions of mainland Portugal and the autonomous regions of Madeira and the Azores, observed that the majority of nurses (89.9%) usually deal with adolescents, 88.5% have no specific training in sexuality, and this training differs from one health sub-region to another. For 95.0% of those surveyed, contraception is the subject they most often talk about, 86.5% suggest that friends are young people's confidants when it comes to sexuality, and 55.4% consider that it is the family who is most responsible for sexual education.

Along these lines, Prazeres, Laranjeira, Marques et al. (2005, p. 23) point out that

As far as hospitals are concerned, the care processes in emergency, inpatient and outpatient departments, generally linked to pediatrics, reveal a remarkable diversity in the models adopted. It is worth mentioning the difficulties that still exist in terms of adapting responses to the characteristics and needs of individuals at these ages, particularly in hospitals with no specific structure/space for adolescents; with regard to professional preparation to respond to individuals at these ages, *it is* mentioned by the patients themselves.

Knowing the changes and characteristics of adolescence can undoubtedly help nurses not only to better understand the experiences of this phase of the life cycle, but also the world of the adolescent in a more global way.

It should be noted that, despite the results presented by Bràs (2008), the changes in the conditions of adolescent socialization are a paradigm that we cannot avoid. One of the typical characteristics of the experience of sexuality in modernity is the radical modification of the communication contexts in which it takes place, in the sense of a saturation of messages on social issues.

A study carried out by Vilar and Ferreira (2009), which covered 2621 adolescents from 63 secondary schools across the country, sought to find out more about the quality, limits, strengths and weaknesses of sexual education for Portuguese adolescents, the role played by schools and other socializing agents, and the impact that better or worse quality sexual education has on adolescents' sexual and preventive behaviour, came to the conclusion that health professionals have the same weight as siblings and other family members as sources of information, always with an average of less than 20%, with the exception of the topic "body changes in adolescence" which, in the specific case of girls, is discussed with the sibling in around 21% of cases. The topic most often discussed with health professionals is "contraception", at around 20%. However, this topic is counterbalanced by rates of around 60% when talking to friends.

Corroborating the previous study is the work carried out by Oliveira (2011) with a sample of 545 adolescents between the ages of 12 and 18 and concludes that the preferred interlocutors for talking about sexuality were friends (58%), 40.9% of adolescents choose their mother, 16.1% their father, 14.7% their girlfriend, 13.8% their siblings, 12.5% their teachers and health technicians are chosen by only 4.6% of adolescents.

The two previous studies relegate the role of the health professional to the background. It is known that the information gathered by adolescents about their sexuality may not be the most feasible from their group of friends or even family, but it can be taken as reliable and lead to dubious behavior. Nurses, as actors in the health system, must play a decisive role in teaching and intervening with adolescents, in order to help them experience their sexuality in an informed, responsible and pleasurable way, with the least risk to their health. Thus, Clemente, Mota and Pacheco (2010) emphasize that it is precisely in this area that nurses play a key role in teaching, welcoming and intervening with adolescents, in order to help them experience their sexuality in an informed and pleasant way, making sure that the adolescent is well looked after and given timely guidance. As a result, there is a need to program a particular form of care aimed at adolescents, such as the adolescent nursing consultation, in order to raise awareness of the need to adopt healthy lifestyles and experience responsible and informed sexuality (Clemente, Mota & Pacheco, 2010).

The healthy development of young people is an important strategic aspect in the life of any community. With this in mind, the national youth health program, a study developed by Prazeres, Laranjeira, Marques et al. (2005: 12) concludes that

Education, prevention, protection and the desirable achievement of health gains are necessary resources for achieving this goal and, from this perspective, the development/health binomial, as mutually determining elements, appears to be inseparable. In this area, what is at stake is not only the current health situation of individuals in the younger age groups, but also what it could become in their future lives - and those of the generations that follow them.

Nursing, as a profession and academic discipline, needs to assert itself in the context of the professions and disciplines that develop with it in the field of health. In order to do this, its ability to focus, intervene and, above all, its social usefulness need to be affirmed and made visible. With this in mind, Bràs (2012), when asking adolescents about the ideal place to talk to health professionals about problems related to their sexuality, concluded that, for 51.9% of girls and 43.9% of boys, the preferred place to talk to health professionals about problems related to sexuality should be the health center. However, 43.7% of girls and 43.3% of boys believe that these professionals should be at school, where they spend most of their time. In the study carried out by Bràs in 2008, 17.9% of the respondents suggested school and other places.

Therefore, the guidance given by the health professional must not be prejudiced, nor supported by moral or religious signs. Appropriate nomenclature should preferably be used, not jargon. Adolescents and their families need to be informed about the physical, biological, emotional and psychosocial transformations at this stage of the adolescent's life cycle and their consequences.

However, the previous study indicates that for 51.9% of girls and 43.9% of boys, the ideal place to talk to health professionals about problems in the sphere of sexuality is the health center. However, the same study indicates that around 17% of young people mention another place to talk about sexuality, and even 43.7% of girls and 43.3% of boys would prefer health professionals to talk to them at school. This must be translated into a close relationship between the various health institutions and the environment outside these institutions.

In this regard, Prazeres, Laranjeira, Marques et al. (2005) conclude that there is a need to reflect more effectively on what is known about adolescents' patterns of use of health institutions. In this area, it is worth mentioning a set of representations by professionals about the profile of contacts with services at this age, insofar as it is commonly considered that adolescents underuse the resources made available to them or do so inappropriately. On the other hand, it is considered that they are reluctant to inform themselves and ask for help from health professionals, and that they are unaware of the type of services on offer. The aforementioned authors also mention that it is common to admit that adolescents fear the attitudes of professionals, namely breaches of confidentiality, that they make the approach to care dependent on previous experiences and that they feel out of place in the services, particularly boys.

Thus, the health professional must be a simplifier who enables adolescents to broaden their ability to judge and accept the decisions of others with whom they interact. Making it possible for adolescents to understand and reveal their perspectives, so that they can accept the feelings, opinions and decisions of others that are different from their own.

When addressing the intervention of nurses in promoting the sexual and reproductive health of adolescents, reference is also made to the premise emanating from Regulation no. 127/2011, of February 18, which states that "nursing care focuses on promoting the health projects that each person lives and pursues" (Preamble). As such, nurses specializing in Maternal, Obstetric and Gynaecological Health Nursing take on autonomous interventions in the target group in their professional practice, promoting quality care that is culturally sensitive and congruent with the needs of the population.

Bearing in mind that sexual and reproductive education should start as early as possible and should be continuous and linked to the education of all children, adolescents and young people, it should be initiated and taken up by parents, complemented by schools and health professionals. It is therefore essential that nurses work on sexuality by promoting young people's self-esteem, whether during individual consultations, in groups or in partnership activities with the community and schools.

According to the Order of Nurses (2010), the issue of sexuality in adolescents is very relevant and topical, and they are a priority group in terms of sexual education, reproductive health and the adoption of healthy lifestyles. In this way, the same organization advocates that the role of nurses should be that of educators, with a view to promoting a responsible, rewarding sexuality that is capable of cooperating in the realization of the young person themselves as a person in all their fullness and in a holistic vision. It's also important to note that many students in higher education are still in their teens, subject to various biological, psychosocial, moral and sexual transformations (Braconnier & Marcelli, 2007). As such, as age advances and nature transforms children into adolescents and young people, the family loses its role as advisor, and it is at school and in the peer group that young people look for information. As they grow up, learning takes place spontaneously, through modeling, primarily in the family and later in the group of friends, and in a more structured way in the community and at school. To intervene in individuals is to intervene in their contexts, and school health is a field par excellence for intervention. That said, nurses must intervene to promote activities that lead to an active lifestyle and reduce risky behaviors and attitudes towards sexuality in young people, emphasizing health promotion and disease prevention measures.

It is indisputable that the path to responsible sexuality involves communication between parents and children, peer groups and health professionals. Thus, health education aims to preserve individual and collective health by equipping students with the knowledge, attitudes and values that will help them make positive and safe choices and adopt more appropriate decisions regarding their sex life. Therefore, the lack of information hinders decision-making and the change of healthy behaviors.

The construction of structured intervention projects in the area of sexuality based on the directives set out in Law No. 60/2009, of August 6, regulated by Ministerial Order No. 196/2010, of April 9, is essential. Nursing intervention in the implementation of dynamic strategies and interventions that engage adolescents more in sexuality issues is also considered relevant, with particular emphasis on the issue of affectivity.

Adolescents need to know more about biological aspects, contraceptive methods and sexually transmitted infections. In addition, this stage of life can make a decisive contribution to achieving identity and autonomy, which will be reflected in adult life. A harmonious and satisfying sexuality becomes a fundamental value in the modern concept of health. Today, it doesn't really make sense to conceive of a state of physical, psychological and social well-being without a fulfilling sex life (Ribeiro & Fernandes, 2009).

Bearing in mind, as Alves (2010) points out, that sexuality is a fundamental aspect of human life, comprising physiological, psychological, social, cultural and spiritual dimensions, and knowing, as already mentioned, that the awakening to sexuality is now increasingly precocious, the consequences of a premature and thoughtless start to adolescent sexual life, combined with vulnerability and risks, with undesirable effects, namely pregnancy and sexually transmitted infections, nurses play a decisive role in intervening with young people, in order to help them experience their sexual and reproductive health in an informed and positive way, ensuring that they are given timely guidance (Oliveira, Carvalho & Silva, 2008).

In this sense, nursing intervention in this area should presuppose effective communication, based on scientific and legal grounds, and an appropriate relationship between nurses and adolescents, by establishing an empathetic and assertive climate of respect, so that they feel safe in their intimacy and privacy, guaranteeing quality in the provision of nursing care and all the ethical guidelines and deontologies inherent to the nursing profession (Oliveira, Carvalho & Silva, 2008). According to the same authors, promoting reproductive and sexual health should be one of the nurses' priorities, particularly in family planning consultations. In the same vein, Flora, Rodrigues and Paiva (2013) argue that a planned intervention in sexual and reproductive education promotes responsible sexuality, which will translate into balance for adolescents, as well as making health services more profitable. The aforementioned authors also see as advantages of this intervention the reduction in cases of sexually transmitted infections and pregnancy in young people, as well as the reduction in the number of terminations of pregnancy and the percentage of pregnancies at these ages.

Although health education is an activity carried out with intent, it leads to health-related learning, generating changes in knowledge and ways of thinking, which is called the process of *empowerment* of populations, whose meaning refers to "inner power", "control" or "self-confidence" (Ramos, 2003). Bearing these assumptions in mind, the notion of *empowerment* is considered to be applicable to the promotion and prevention of adolescents' sexual and reproductive health, insofar as it is a continuous and multidimensional process that takes place in a specific *location*, characterized by psychological, cultural and economic dimensions, where adolescents acquire the confidence to understand their situation and increase their control over factors that may put their sexual and reproductive health at risk. Thus, and taking into account what Ramos (2003) says, in terms of promoting and preventing sexual and reproductive health, *empowerment* is a process that allows adolescents to gain greater control over their decisions and actions that may affect their health.

It should also be noted that Ramos (2003) distinguished four fundamental factors in an *empowerment* process: access to information, i.e. adolescents who are correctly informed about sexual and reproductive health are better prepared to exercise their rights and acquire opportunities; inclusion and participation, which refer to opportunities to participate in decision-making; responsibility and organizational capacity, insofar as adolescents are subject to numerous ecological transitions, both in and out of school, and mobilize resources to deal with everyday problems.

Sexual and reproductive health is an area in which psychological and social factors, namely the perception of "social norms" and the "modeling of behavior", such as the adoption of models established by peers, play a key role. With regard, by way of example, to protective behaviors, namely condom use, conversations about safe sex and HIV testing, according to Matos et al. (2011), it is adolescents who have not had sex education at school who have a negative attitude towards these protective behaviors. As you can see, it's difficult to try to change the behavior of adolescents if you don't really want to change: education helps people to generate the strength that will support them in making decisions, in other words, and in line with Pender's Health Protection Model, you have to check whether previous behavior and the characteristics inherited from the environment and acquired influence and/or affect the regulation of current behavior in terms of promoting sexual and reproductive health, in this specific case. Change only occurs when it awakens meaning and the desire to open up to new experiences. However, real change is not an easy process; it always involves autonomy, motivation and decision-making (Reis & Matos, 2008).

According to Matos et al. (2011), knowledge does not necessarily lead to preventive behavior. They are responsible for developing the skills that lead to preventive sexual behavior. Therefore, safe sexual behavior doesn't just depend on the presence of knowledge. It depends on the motivation to perform preventive behaviors and the skills needed to carry them out. This process implies, according to Noler (1996, cited by Tomey & Alliggod, 2011), that adolescents also commit to behaviors that allow them to anticipate benefits in terms of sexual and reproductive health. Perceived competence or self-efficacy to perform a certain behavior increases the likelihood of commitment to the action and the actual performance of the behavior (Tomey & Alliggod, 2011).

In short, the learning process takes place formally and informally, with contradictions and conflicting messages between the various actors. But it's important to note that the formal is not opposed to the informal, they just coexist. The role of health professionals and nurses in particular, as actors in formal learning, is very important because they are professionals of reference: a health professional is believed much more than a friend, television or the internet, or even a parent.

PART II - EMPIRICAL STUDY

CHAPTER III - METHODOLOGICAL FRAMEWORK

This chapter describes the methodological procedures inherent in the empirical study, starting with the theoretical conceptualization of the object of study, the research question and respective objectives, the research model and type of study, the selection of participants, the description of the data collection instrument, ethical and formal aspects and the analysis of the data, where the methodology followed is specified.

1. RESEARCH QUESTIONS AND OBJECTIVES

The elaboration of the research question(s) is the phase that should enhance knowledge of the phenomenon under study in a meaningful way (Polit & Hungler, 2004).

With this in mind, we came up with the following research question:

- What attitudes do nurses working in Primary Health Care have towards adolescent sexuality?

Defining objectives is essentially about answering questions such as "for what?" and "for whom?", and they must be rational, relevant, concrete, realistic, unequivocal and measurable (Fortin, 2009). As such, the same author states that the objectives should provide answers to the problem formulated, as well as clarifying the central research question.

It is therefore imperative to contextualize and define the objectives of this work. The objectives of this study were therefore:

- To know which age groups most often seek health services for sexual issues/problems;

- To find out which sexes of adolescents go to health centers the most;

- To see if the reasons why adolescents go to the health center are the same for both sexes, and if not, what the differences are;

- To know the risk situations in terms of adolescents' sexual and reproductive health that appear most frequently in adolescent care;

- To find out about the sexual content most frequently approached by adolescents;

- To find out how nurses rate their comfort/discomfort in dealing with sexual content;

- To find out what nurses think about sexual relationships between adolescents;

- To find out what nurses think about the age of sexual initiation;

- To see how sexual orientation issues (homosexual, heterosexual, bisexual, transsexual) appear in adolescent care and how nurses usually deal with them;

- To find out whether nurses also address issues related to affections, feelings and emotional relationships in their approach to sexual matters with adolescents, what kind of issues arise, whether they differ between boys and girls and how nurses address them;

-	To see how nurses assess the level of knowledge and information that adolescents have on issues related to sexuality;

-	To find out whether there are different levels of information and knowledge among young people, whether there are differences between boys and girls;

-	erify how nurses classify adolescents' access to health services in the area of sexual and reproductive health;

-	To know the real importance of nurses in responding to adolescents in terms of sexual and reproductive health;

-	To see how the promotion of sexual health in adolescence can contribute (or not) to the overall well-being of adolescents now and in the future.

2. SAMPLE AND ITS CHARACTERISTICS

Non-probabilistic convenience sampling was used to select the participants. Given the scope and objectives of the study, we wanted to gather information from nurses who work directly with adolescents. Therefore, we sought to hear the opinion of the professionals most directly involved in intervening with adolescents and agreeing to take part in the study voluntarily, which were the criteria for inclusion in the sample. The criteria for including the subjects in the sample were based on what Morse (1998, cited in Flick, 2005) defines as "good informants": subjects who have the necessary knowledge and experience of the subject or object in question. They must also have the capacity for reflection and articulation, the time to be questioned and the willingness to participate. If all these premises are met, the subject meets all the conditions to be included in the study and their inclusion is defined as "primary Morse selection".

According to Freixo (2011, p. 182), a sample "is made up of a group of subjects taken from a population, with sampling consisting of a set of operations that make it possible to choose a group of subjects or any other representative element of the population studied". Thus, the target population consists of 163 nurses up to December 31, 2015, working in 14 Health Centers, and 1 Health Center was excluded because it refused to participate in the study. The sample therefore consisted of 49 nurses interviewed, representing 30% of the target population. It should be noted that the head nurse of each Health Center was contacted and asked to interview the nurses who have the most contact with adolescents, so those proposed were interviewed, as shown in Table 1:

Table 2 - Distribution of nurses interviewed by Health Center

Health Centers	No. of nurses interviewed
Seia	4
Gouveia	4
Trancoso	3
Figueira	3
Riverside	8
Guard	1

Meda	3
Pinhel	4
Butters	1
Ovens	4
Sabugal	3
Almeida	8
Trancoso	3
Total	**49**

With regard to the sociodemographic and professional characterization of the sample interviewed (n=49), it can be said that the majority of the sample is made up of nurses (92.0%), which corroborates data from the Order of Nurses (2015), according to which, in 2013, 81.7% of nurses were registered with the Order of Nurses. The age data shows that nurses have a minimum age of 21 and a maximum age of 54, corresponding to an average age of 43.54 years, with a standard deviation of 8.33 years. Nurses are on average older (=44.00 years±7.055 years) than nurses (=43.37 years±9.174 years). The data on length of service shows that nurses have a minimum of 0.5 months' service and a maximum of 32 years, corresponding to an average length of service of 20.49 years with a standard deviation of 6.512 years. In general, the length of service corresponds to the length of service at the current Health Center.

3. Techniques USED

One of the most important decisions to be made by the researcher is the type of research, always bearing in mind the state of knowledge regarding the problem to be studied, not forgetting that the type of study is in line with the questions and hypotheses formulated, thus serving to answer them.

There are therefore two main types of research: qualitative research and quantitative research (Lobiondo-Wood & Haber, 2001).

The type of study followed in this work will be qualitative, a method considered by Bogdan and Bikklen (1994) to be humanistic, because when researchers study subjects in a qualitative way they try to get to know them as people and experience what they experience in their daily lives (they don't reduce words and actions to statistical equations). Researchers are more interested in the research process than just the results or products that come out of it. According to these authors, in qualitative research, the research plan is flexible.

Bogdan and Biklen (1994, p. 132) present the five main characteristics of qualitative research:

1.   The natural situation is the source of the data, and the researcher is the key instrument for data collection;

2.   Your first concern is to describe and only secondarily to analyze the data;

3.   The key issue is the whole process, i.e. what happened, as well as the product and the end result;

4.   The data is analyzed intuitively, as if all the parts of a jigsaw puzzle were put together;

5.   It essentially concerns the meaning of things, i.e. the 'why' and the 'what'.

The same authors state that the aim is to collect data in the natural environment in which the actions take place, to describe the situations experienced by the participants and to interpret the meanings they attribute to them -

in this case, the attitude of nurses working in Primary Health Care towards adolescent sexuality - which justifies the use of a qualitative approach.

In qualitative research, interviews can be used in two ways. They can be the dominant strategy for data collection or they can be used in conjunction with participant observation, document analysis and other techniques. In all these situations, the interview is used to collect descriptive data in the subject's own language, allowing the researcher to intuitively develop an idea of how subjects interpret aspects of the world (Bogdan & Biklen, 1994, p.134).

Qualitative research is "descriptive" and must be rigorous and derive directly from the data collected. Data includes interview transcripts, observation records, written documents (personal and official), among others. The researchers analyze the data collected, respecting, as far as possible, the form in which it was recorded or transcribed (Bogdan & Bikklen, 1994). In this type of study, according to the same authors, the researcher is the "instrument" of data collection; the validity and reliability of the data depends very much on their sensitivity, knowledge and experience. The question of the researcher's objectivity is the main problem in qualitative research, where the central concern is not whether the results can be generalized, but whether other contexts and subjects can be generalized to them.

These were the guiding principles followed in carrying out this study, namely: the use of interviews. The answers obtained through the interviews were subjected to content analysis according to the principles of Bardin (2004).

The term "content analysis" refers to "a set of techniques for analyzing communications in order to obtain, by means of systematic and objective procedures for describing the content of messages, indicators (quantitative or not) that allow the inference of knowledge relating to the conditions of production/reception (inferred variables) of these messages" (Bardin, 2004, p. 47).

According to the same author, it consists of a methodological technique that can be applied to a variety of discourses and all forms of communication, whatever the nature of their medium. In this analysis, the researcher seeks to understand the characteristics, structures or models behind the fragments of messages taken into consideration. Bardin (2004) indicates that the use of content analysis involves three fundamental phases: pre-analysis, exploration of the material and treatment of the results - inference and interpretation, which are the steps followed in this work.

Below is a summary of the categories and subcategories that emerged from the registration units of the nurses interviewed (see Table 2).

Table 3 - Summary of categories and subcategories

Categories	Sub-categories
Ethnic groups that most often seek health services for sexual issues/problems	14-18 years 15-18 years 18-21 years
Who goes to the health center most often?	Boys

	Girls
	Boys and girls
Reasons why adolescents go to the health center	Pregnancy
	Contraceptive methods
	Sexually transmitted infections
Risk situations in terms of adolescents' sexual and reproductive health that appear most frequently in adolescent care	Termination of pregnancy Contraceptive methods
Sexual content most frequently addressed by adolescents	Sexually transmitted infections
	Contraceptive methods
Classification of comfort/discomfort when dealing with sexual content	Totally comfortable
	Comfortable - 4 on a scale of 1 to 5
Nurses' attitudes towards sexual relationships among adolescents	Positive attitude
Age for starting sex	There's no age to start having sex
How sexual orientation issues (homosexual, heterosexual, bisexual, transsexual) appear in adolescent care	Infrequent questions about homosexual, bisexual and transsexual orientation
Addressing issues related to adolescents' affections, feelings and affective relationships	Teenagers don't directly address issues of affection
Assessment of the level of knowledge and information adolescents have on issues related to sexuality	Teenagers have misinformation
Adolescents' access to sexual reproductive health services	Rating of 1 Very difficult
	Rating 4/5 Very easy
The real importance of nurses in responding to adolescents in sexual reproductive health	A lot of importance
How adolescent sexual health promotion may (or may not) contribute to the overall well-being of adolescents now and in the future	Contributes to the promotion of present and future well-being

4. DATA COLLECTION INSTRUMENT

4.1. THE INTERVIEW

To obtain the necessary data, a semi-structured interview was used (see Appendix II). The interview is used to collect descriptive data "in the subject's own language, allowing the researcher to intuitively develop an idea of how subjects interpret aspects of the world" (Bogdan & Biklen, 1994, p. 134).

Within social research, the interview is characterized as a tool used to collect data (Lakatos & Marconi, 2004).

According to the same authors, the desired information is obtained in particular with the help of an interview script which should contain a list of items listed and defined in advance, based on a central problem.

Lakatos and Marconi (2004) point out that in the semi-structured interview, unlike the structured interview, the interviewer is free to progress in any situation to whatever destination he or she deems necessary, which is a way of analyzing a broader horizon of a given question. Normally, the questions are open-ended and allow for answers that fit into an informal dialog and are perfectly acceptable. This type of interview can be defined as a method for obtaining data that presupposes a constant dialog involving the interviewee and the interviewer, who must coordinate this dialog based on their objectives. Based on this premise, interest is focused exclusively on what can add pertinent information to the research context (Lakatos & Marconi, 2004).

The interview used in this study consists of a set of questions that allow us to draw up a sociodemographic and professional profile of the nurses and questions that allow us to find out their attitudes towards adolescent sexuality, as shown below.

The first part contains 6 individual characterization questions, namely: age, gender, educational qualifications, length of service, length of service in the current Health Center and professional category. The second part is made up of a set of 14 open questions to gather information on nurses' attitudes towards adolescent sexuality.

4.2. ETHICAL CONSIDERATIONS

For the interviews to be carried out, a formal request for authorization was made to the Health Ethics Committee of the Guarda Local Health Unit (cf. Appendix III) so that the interviews could be carried out in the following Health Centers: Almeida Health Center, Fornos de Algodres Health Center, Gouveia Health Center, Guarda Health Center, Meda Health Center, "A Ribeirinha" Local Health Unit, Manteigas Health Center, Pinhel Health Center, Sabugal Health Center, Seia Health Center, Vila Nova de Foz Côa Health Center and Figueira de Castelo Rodrigo Health Center.

The interviews were carried out freely and conscientiously, without any physical, psychological, moral or deceptive coercion, which prevented the nurses who took part in the study from freely expressing their personal will, which meant that each interviewee was given a request for informed consent. Before the interviews took place, we described the objectives to each interviewee and guaranteed the confidentiality of the data. Clarification was guaranteed and they were informed of their choice to participate voluntarily and freely in the study.

It should also be noted that, in order to guarantee the confidentiality of each interviewee, we assigned them a code when processing their testimonies, for example E1 (interviewee 1).

CHAPTER IV - ANALYSIS AND DISCUSSION OF RESULTS

1. ANALYSIS OF INTERVIEW DATA

The results are then presented, taking into account the research question and the objectives outlined. After their presentation, a discussion takes place based on the literature review.

1.1. AGE GROUPS THAT MOST OFTEN SEEK HEALTH SERVICES FOR HEALTH ISSUES/PROBLEMS

Table 4 shows the results for category 1 - *Age groups who most often seek health services for sexual issues/problems*. According to 29 informants, the age group of adolescents who most *often* seek these services is 14-18 years old, 11 nurses mentioned the 15-18 age group and 9 indicated the 18-21 age group. It is also important to note that some nurses mentioned another age group, from 10 to 18 years old. However, these adolescents do not go to the Health Center of their own free will or on the advice of their parents, but because they are called for a comprehensive examination, and they go accompanied by their parents.

"Adolescents don't go to the health center for free, but they are called in for a comprehensive examination (...)" (E23)

"As far as I can tell, there are few, if any, teenagers who come to us, but the few who do, usually come by invitation." (E4).

"(...) there isn't much demand from young people, perhaps because of inhibition or because they're looking for information elsewhere, on the internet, from other colleagues. What is certain *is* that demand *is* relatively small (.)" (E11).

Other nurses also referred to this age group not as adolescents who might go to the Health Center for sexuality issues, but in a school context, with nurses going to meet them more in schools and not the other way around. This contact is made in the classroom and/or in the student's office:

"(...) adolescents don't often come to the health center to talk about sexuality either, perhaps because they feel inhibited, or because when we go to school, we talk about sexuality (...) often this contact is made in the student's office, where they talk about contraception and sexually transmitted diseases (...)" (E15).

"The ones we intervene with the most are more at school health level (...)" (E17).

"(...) now we don't intervene in the health center, it's more at school level, only in the classroom or in the student's office (...) we make the office more dynamic with the question of food and the children are invited to go. Now it's like this, sexuality issues come up after the classroom sessions and they often go to the student's office to ask questions they didn't want to ask in the classroom in front of their classmates (...)" (E9).

Table 4 - Age groups most frequently seeking health services for sexual issues/problems

Category	Sub-categories	Frequency
Age groups that most often seek health services for sexual issues/problems	14-18 years	29
	15-18 years	11
	18-21 years	9

1.2. WHO GOES TO THE HEALTH CENTER MOST OFTEN

Table 5 shows the results for category 2 - *Who goes to the health center most often* - from which three subcategories emerged. It emerged that 34 of the nurses interviewed said that girls most often seek health services because of sexual issues/problems, which, according to them, could be explained by the fact that they are nurses and boys don't feel as comfortable:

"(.) it's the girls, because maybe we're nurses and they feel more at ease (.")" which is the opposite, according to the 4 nurses interviewed, because the demand, in their case, is predominantly from boys (.)" (E22).

"It's more the guys who are looking, maybe because they're nurses, they don't feel so inhibited. Even in conversations with other colleagues, they say exactly the opposite: they're the ones looking. Maybe they come and discreetly try to find out who's on duty - I assume that's why. I can say that the people who come to us are always male... for me, the people who come to us are in the 16-18 age group and they are almost always male." (E12).

It was also found that 11 of the nurses interviewed said that there was a demand for these services from adolescents of both sexes:

"Demand, although it's low, when they come they're from both sexes (.)" (E15).

However, most of the nurses said that there was very little demand for this at the health center, which could be due to two reasons: on the one hand, there aren't many adolescents in the more rural areas; on the other hand, the cultural issue prevails:

E32 "They won't because it's a cultural issue".

"The cultural issue and prejudice because Sabugal is an imminently rural area" (E19).

They consider that sexuality is present in all age groups, but parents don't recognize this and most of them don't feel comfortable enough to encourage their children and don't see the approach to this subject as natural in relation to other subjects:

"Sexuality is something that is present in all age groups, but parents don't recognize it and most of them don't feel comfortable with it and don't see the approach to this subject as something natural in relation to other subjects." (E17)

Cultural issues and prejudice continue to prevail, especially in rural areas. One nurse said

"Often, not going to the health center is also due to the fact that adolescents look for other means of information, such as the internet and their peers, highlighting the inhibition factor" (E10).

Table 5 - Who goes most often to the Health Center

Category	Sub-categories	Response indicators	Frequency
Who goes to the health center most often?	Boys	Boys because they feel more comfortable with a nurse	4
	Girls	Girls because they feel more comfortable with a nurse	34
	Boys and girls	Both seek health services	11

1.3.   REASONS WHY ADOLESCENTS GO TO THE HEALTH CENTER

According to the results, and with regard to the reasons why adolescents go to the Health Center, all the interviewees mentioned that it is common for adolescents of both sexes to go to the Health Center because of contraceptive methods. Twenty-seven nurses said that the majority of girls also seek information about unwanted pregnancies, while 15 nurses said that adolescents seek information about sexually transmitted infections (see Table 6). Some nurses said that adolescents in the 18-21 age group seek health services, especially girls, because of pregnancy termination and contraceptive issues, while very few boys do so, delegating this responsibility to the girls:

"(...) They almost always come to us because of unwanted pregnancies or contraceptive methods to avoid pregnancy. They don't discuss the question of affections with the nurses, they don't come to us for that at all. It's a complex subject (.)" (E12);

"(.) they come to us more because of contraceptive methods to avoid unwanted pregnancies (.)" (E9).

They pointed out that, in some cases, teenagers go to the nurses in the student office at school to get contraceptive methods, particularly the pill for girls.

Table 6 - Reasons why adolescents go to the health center

Category	Sub-categories	Response indicators	Frequency
Reasons why adolescents go to the health center	Pregnancy	Girls want to ask questions about unwanted pregnancy - prevention - the pill and the morning after pill	27
	Contraceptive methods	Both boys and girls are looking for contraceptive methods	49
	Sexually transmitted infections	Both boys and girls seek information about sexually transmitted infections	15

With regard to the risk situations in terms of adolescents' sexual reproductive health that appear most frequently in adolescent care, as shown in Table 7, the search for contraceptive methods essentially by girls (n=49) stands out, followed by voluntary termination of pregnancy, which was considered by 11 nurses to be a borderline situation:

"(...) sometimes they look for a reason to start contraception, for example condoms, because they don't seek this information from their parents and then there's the difficulty of going to the family doctor or a doctor who can make this assessment and prescribe (...)" (E24);

"(...) they look more for contraception and then there have been a few situations of unprotected relationships in which the method failed for some reason and they needed our help to refer them (.)" (E11);

"(...) in the little bit that they see, I always try my best to address the issues of sexuality, to find out what's behind it, but they come more because of contraceptive methods in the sense of an unwanted pregnancy (.)" (E12).

Table 7 - Risk situations in terms of adolescents' sexual and reproductive health that appear most frequently in adolescent care

Category	Sub-categories	Response indicators	Frequency
Risk situations in terms of adolescents' sexual and reproductive health that appear most frequently in adolescent care	Termination of pregnancy	Girls on the edge - voluntary termination of pregnancy	12
	Contraceptive methods	Search for contraceptive methods, especially among girls.	49

1.4. SEXUAL CONTENT MOST FREQUENTLY ADDRESSED BY ADOLESCENTS

The topics most frequently addressed by adolescents continue to be contraception (n=49) and, to a lesser extent, issues related to sexually transmitted infections (n=12) (see Table 8). One nurse said that when:

"(...) the whole team goes to school, there is more concern on the part of adolescents about these sexual issues (...)" (E13).

However, it has to be said that the majority of nurses say that they don't go out into the community to talk to adolescents about school health, and this is a gap that *cuts* across most of the health centers studied.

In this context, it is important to note that the majority of nurses mentioned that adolescents do not talk or seek information about love and relationship issues:

"Sexually transmitted diseases, means of contraception, the affective part of a love relationship, because we've seen that, especially in adolescence, this affective part is increasingly undervalued, they don't recognize this importance and this aspect which is decisive. It's very important because teenagers are in peer groups at this stage and there's always the influence of one on the other and then there's pressure - I did it, that one did it too and if I don't do it I'm not as good as him and I'm not at his level" (E 25).

There was a prevailing view that adolescents don't address love and relationship issues of their own volition, and that this is a topic that is rarely dealt with, and when it is, it's at the urging of the nurses, who consider it to be a more complex subject. On the other hand, the majority of nurses pointed out that adolescents see them more as a source of information, considering the issue of affections to be a subject to be dealt with by a psychologist:

"(.) They don't approach the question of affections, they feel ashamed, and they see nurses more as a sense of information about diseases. And it also has to do with the way we approach them, we don't talk about affections (.) (E22);

"(.) Affections for them are more about the psychologist (.)" (E32);

"(...) I don't want to make that judgment, but I can say that if there is a question of affections, they don't discuss it with us. It's not an easy subject to tackle either. Basically, their problem isn't their affections, but talking to us. If they look for help, they look for help other than us (.)" (E12).

Nonetheless, the importance of the approach to affections was a common theme in the nurses' testimonies, and one nurse even mentioned it:

"(...) this could be a prophylactic means of preventing violence in dating and adult life" (E32).

The vast majority said that it was important to convey to teenagers the idea of knowing how to contextualize sexual intercourse in the context of the relationship, encouraging trust between the couple, as well as making teenagers aware that they are dealing with a stable partner, whether the sexual relationship is meaningful, whether, in the case of girls, they are pressured into having sex, whether there is any manifestation of violence in the relationship. The opinion of the nurses stood out, who said that for most adolescents what matters is having sex, which is a manifestation of the pressure from society to start having sex between the ages of 14-15, in other words, there is an anticipation of the start of sexual life without any kind of contextualization in terms of love and relationship issues, leading adolescents to understand this natural dimension of human life.

The vast majority of nurses consider the approach to affections to be extremely important:

"(...) it's important that we approach affections with young people from a perspective of being able to listen without expressions of scandal or modesty, of getting adolescents to reflect on their right to pleasure, helping them to realize that this right to pleasure is greater the greater the aspects of affection it encompasses, helping them to realize that the "promotion" of the adult, which every adolescent desires, is not obtained through the consummation of a merely mechanical and often traumatizing sexual relationship" (E22).

Ultimately:

"(.) to provide correct and rigorous information about sexuality, which should be seen as a human condition and experienced in a pleasurable way, so that the decision, whatever it may be, is a conscious one (.) (E15).

The reality, in the opinion of the nurses interviewed, is that:

"(...) adolescents don't have a true understanding of the question of affections in sexuality, also because they don't have a fixed dating relationship (...)" (E5);

"(...) moving from tide to tide, without covering the whole ocean", in other words, in temporal terms, the relationships are short-lived, becoming more physical than properly affectionate (...) (E11).

When nurses talk about affections, they focus on the issue of violence, respect for others, and the need for a healthy relationship. According to the nurses, the lack of initiative on the part of the adolescents in wanting to talk about love and relationships is a problem.

"(...) a reflection of the very lack of affection that many adolescents show, particularly in relation to friendships that are very virtual, manifesting behaviors of internet addiction and becoming very mechanized" (E23).

In this respect, they think there should be, according to one nurse:

"(.) greater intervention on the part of the school, including training for parents on the importance of affections in their children's sexuality (.)" (E9).

In this sense, one of the nurses interviewed stated that:

"(...) there is a notorious lack of dialog between parents and children, due to the parents' professional lives, leaving them no room for dialog about sexuality (..)" (E28).

Table 8 - Sexual content most frequently addressed by adolescents

Category	Sub-categories	Response indicators	Frequency
Sexual content most frequently addressed by adolescents	Sexually transmitted infections	Girls on the edge - voluntary termination of pregnancy	12
	Contraceptive methods	Questions about, for example, putting on a condom, taking the pill.	49

1.5. CLASSIFICATION OF COMFORT/DISCOMFORT WHEN DEALING WITH SEXUAL CONTENT

The nurses were asked to rate their comfort/discomfort with each of the sexual topics they discuss with adolescents on a scale of 1 to 5 (where 1 is "Total discomfort" and 5 is "Totally comfortable"). As shown in Table 9, 37 of the interviewees rated their comfort at the maximum point on the scale, justifying this total comfort with the importance of prioritizing these topics with adolescents:

"(...) Totally comfortable. It's very difficult to work with them sometimes, but I feel I'm open enough to talk. But they don't come to us. We have a youth support office, but the demand is residual" (E22).

However, some nurses said that

"(...) sometimes it's very difficult to work with them, but they feel open to talk (...)" (E40).

For these nurses,

"(...) sexuality is a topic like any other, with the same importance as any other health topic and it comes up as naturally as any other topic (...)" (E17).

However, they feel that they have to come up with appropriate strategies to get around the problems that arise.

It was also noted that 12 nurses rated their comfort in talking to adolescents about sexuality at point 4 on the scale, justifying this rating with the fact that adolescents often feel inhibited when talking about their affections:

"(...) *the* problem is that teenagers often feel inhibited and don't talk openly, they just seek contraception (...)" (E10);

"(...) I rate it a 4, because there's always one situation or another that makes us more embarrassed...but as a general rule, because we've been doing this for a while, the questions they ask we know how to answer...but if there's a question we don't know how to answer, we direct them to the student's office or we tell them that when they come again, we'll try to give them the answer, through the PES teacher") (E23).

Table 9 - Classification of comfort/discomfort in approaching sexual content

Category	Sub-categories	Response indicators	Frequency
Classification of comfort/discomfort in dealing with sexual content	Totally comfortable	They feel completely comfortable approaching sexual content, rating this comfort at the highest point on the scale (5) - openness to talking to adolescents.	37
	Comfortable - 4 on a scale of 1 to 5	On a scale of 1 to 5, rate their comfort in dealing with sexual content at 4, due to the teenagers' own inhibitions.	12

1.6. NURSES' ATTITUDES TOWARDS SEXUAL RELATIONSHIPS AMONG ADOLESCENTS

It was found that all nurses have a positive attitude towards sexual relationships between adolescents, considering that they should understand that life is made up of relationships, which have to be made responsibly and protected, that adolescents should experiment in order to know how to choose the right partner (see Table 10). Nurses also pointed out:

"(...) adolescents first have to discover their own bodies, so that sexuality can occur naturally, but they also have to be "equipped" with a strong repository of affection, know how to distinguish between a relationship of friendship and a relationship with more affection, know how to live this feeling, have a sense of whether it's the right time for sexual intercourse, know how to live their sexual life pleasurably and responsibly (...)" (E22);

"(...) it's important to know how to distinguish between passion and love, as the majority are motivated by passion, which results in sexual relations in a relationship that ends up being short-lived (...)" (E14).

It's important to note that some interviewees reinforced the idea that they don't have a large group of teenagers who come to them and pass on the issue of sexual intercourse itself, which is due to the fact that these are eminently rural areas:

"(...) Here, as I said earlier, we don't have a large group of teenagers who come to us and pass on the question of the sexual act itself" (E12).

Table 10 - Nurses' attitudes towards sexual relationships between adolescents

Category	Sub-categories	Response indicators	Frequency
Nurses' attitudes towards sexual relationships among adolescents	Positive attitude	Life is made up of relationships Relationships have to be done responsibly and protected They must experiment in order to know how to choose Discovery, first and foremost, of the body itself Need to have a strong repository of affection Know how to distinguish between a relationship of friendship and a relationship with more affection, knowing how to live this feeling Know when the time is right for sexual intercourse Know how to live sexual life pleasurably and responsibly Knowing how to distinguish between passion and love	49

1.7. AGE TO START SEX LIFE

Another result that emerged was that all the nurses (n=49) believe that there is no proper age for adolescents to start their sex life (see Table 11), arguing that it should be done responsibly, which also implies that adolescents should decide and not because of social pressure, without letting themselves be led by the stereotype of the media, which suggests that adolescents should start their sex life at the age of 14:

"I wouldn't say there's an age, as long as the person feels comfortable both with themselves and with their partner, it's a normal thing to come up with, it's part of human development and it's normal to come up with it at this time, once you've discovered all these aspects. It's more than normal. Now it's a question of being prepared for it and knowing what you're doing" (E13).

According to one nurse, in view of the stipulation of an age for starting sex at 14, he said that

"(...) there are cases in which adolescents in the 15-16 age group who have not yet started sex feel enormous pressure, feeling that they are already two years too late. This kind of information leads young people to anticipate sexual intercourse, which usually happens under pressure and without being contextualized in a relationship of affection (.)" (E22);

"(...) they are often pressured, because they often hear "that one did it and you haven't done it yet" (E40).

"There's a lot of pressure these days for sexuality to start earlier and earlier and I think young people are taking it in their stride. I mean, everyone has done it except me. So they have to have it at all costs, no matter with whom, and that's why they start earlier and earlier. Society itself sells it to them. When they hear the news that the age at which sexuality begins is 14, they feel this pressure... oh boy, I'm two years too late. This kind of information puts pressure on young people to start sex earlier (...) it gives me the impression that they're going to have this relationship not out of affection, but because of pressure from society" (E22).

This nurse is also of the opinion that

"(...) nurses need to send out a clearer message on this subject, bearing in mind that relationships today are short-lived, unstable, there is an increase in unwanted pregnancies, an increase in the number of abortions, aided by their legalization. There are social ideas that put pressure on them, not out of affection, but out of pressure from society and even masculinity" (E22).

They are of the opinion that they should only start their sex life as long as they feel comfortable both with themselves and with their partner, with E8 mentioning

"(...) it's a perfectly normal event, an integral part of human development and it's normal for it to arise at this time, since it's the stage of discovering all these aspects (...)" (E8).

Their speeches reveal that this should be a rewarding experience, not a trauma for the first time, but a positive memory, lived responsibly. The question lies in the opinion of the interviewees, as one nurse put it:

"(...) whether or not adolescents are ready to start their sex life, which requires nurses to put them in context, relieve them of the pressure that is affecting them, getting to the point and not remedying it, as is usually done (...)" (E16).

On the other hand, it is important, even from the perspective of some nurses, as exemplified by the speech of another nurse:

"(.) to help adolescents sort through the wealth of information they have about sexuality, because not all of it is correct, leading them to inconsequential acts (.)" (E26).

Table 11 - Age of first sexual intercourse

Category	Sub-categories	Response indicators	Frequency
Age for starting sex	There's no age to start having sex	There is no age to start having sex Beginning a sexual life should be done responsibly It's the teenagers who have to decide. More should be done to implement comprehensive sex education in schools, involving affections, and there should be no age stipulation. You have to put teenagers in context. Take the pressure off teenagers. To get to the point and not to patch things up, as usual Teenagers need to feel comfortable Viewing sexuality as a human and natural condition, without age stereotypes Screening information on sexuality Society "sells" adolescents a stereotype of the beginning of sexual life - social pressure It must be a very rewarding experience for teenagers	49

		Let it not be a traumatic experience, but a positive one	

1.8. HOW ISSUES OF SEXUAL ORIENTATION (HOMOSEXUAL, HETEROSEXUAL, BISEXUAL, TRANSSEXUAL) APPEAR IN ADOLESCENT CARE

According to the findings, there are almost no situations in which issues of sexual orientation (homosexual, heterosexual, bisexual, transsexual) are addressed in adolescent care, with 9 nurses even stating that these issues are not part of the content of actions in the school context, and only come up occasionally by some adolescents during sessions (see Table 12). Most of the nurses admitted that girls are more uninhibited, as one of them pointed out:

"(...) the girls end up being more uninhibited when it comes to discussing their sexual orientation, probably because they're talking to a nurse, while the boys are mostly inhibited when it comes to this subject (...)" (E15).

Table 12 - How sexual orientation issues (homosexual, heterosexual, bisexual, transsexual) appear in adolescent care

Category	Sub-categories	Response indicators	Frequency
How sexual orientation issues (homosexual, heterosexual, bisexual, transsexual) appear in adolescent care	Infrequent questions about homosexual, bisexual and transsexual orientation	Adolescents don't address sexual orientation issues Lack of approach to affections Nurses do not address sexual orientation issues directly Teenagers are very introverted when it comes to these issues. Some girls are more open to talking about sexual orientation issues.	49

1.9. ADDRESSING ISSUES RELATED TO ADOLESCENTS' AFFECTIONS, FEELINGS AND AFFECTIVE RELATIONSHIPS

According to the nurses' testimonies (n=49), and as mentioned above, when issues related to adolescents' affections, feelings and relationships are addressed, it is done by the nurses and not by the adolescents (see Table 13), and the topic is introduced discreetly, as most adolescents are not receptive to this subject and do not share their experience of sexuality as a whole with the nurses, as one interviewee put it:

"(...) just looking for contraceptive methods and doubts about unwanted pregnancies (...)" (E37).

Most nurses consider it important to be able to show adolescents that:

"(.) they shouldn't experience sexuality as an isolated act, that it shouldn't be practiced with just anyone, that it should be experienced on the basis of responsibility, trust between partners (.)" (E42).

Table 13 - Approach to questions related to adolescents' affections, feelings and affective relationships

Category	Sub-categories	Response indicators	Frequency
Addressing issues related to adolescents' affections, feelings and affective relationships	Adolescents don't directly address issues of affection	Adolescents don't associate affections with sexuality Adolescents don't discuss their affections with nurses They look for contraceptive methods to prevent unwanted pregnancies	49

| | | Actions in schools do not focus on affections | |
| | | Teenagers don't talk about emotional relationships, they restrict themselves to the physical component | |

1.10. ASSESSMENT OF THE LEVEL OF KNOWLEDGE AND INFORMATION ADOLESCENTS HAVE ON ISSUES RELATED TO SEXUALITY

Based on the speeches of the nurses interviewed, it was found that a significant group believes that the majority of adolescents have misinformation about sexuality (see Table 14), which, in the opinion of one nurse, makes it difficult to understand.

"(...) it's important to help them sort through this information, which almost always comes from the internet or peer groups, so that they can experience their sexuality in a healthy way, from a holistic viewpoint (...)" (E22).

Also according to a nurse:

"Friends are the most sought after by adolescents when they feel the need to clarify their sexuality, because they feel more at ease and have their trust/understanding (.)" (E25).

According to one of the nurses interviewed

"A significant number of adolescents have information in an unresponsible way, because they don't take care to perceive it, without seeking to know what is scientifically correct" (E33).

On the other hand, as one of the interviewees said

"(...) it's important that family nurses take the stance of telling parents that from a certain age their children have to go to the appointment on their own, as parents are an inhibiting factor, which also results in inhibition on the part of nurses to address sexuality as a whole" (E44).

It was also made clear that there are currently no major differences between boys and girls in terms of information,

"(...) both seek information about sexuality in their own way, and girls don't have the traditional format of chastity until marriage, as in the past, which comes from the emancipation of women (.) (E23).

They believe that there is a lot of access to information and if nurses don't distinguish between what is correct and what is not, there is a risk that adolescents will not be experiencing healthy sexuality. Teenagers therefore need to be helped

"(...) sorting out what *is* health promotion from what isn't, which is the primary role of the nurse, especially the family nurse, which means that adolescents have to go to the appointment on their own, because, most of the time, their doubts aren't answered because their parents aren't receptive to these issues, and it's still a taboo" (E39).

Table 14 - Assessment of the degree of knowledge and information adolescents have on issues related to sexuality

Category	Sub-categories	Response indicators	Frequency
Assessment of the level of knowledge and information that	Teenagers have misinformation	Most teenagers have misinformation about sexuality It's important for teenagers to be able to sort through	49

| | | information | |
| | | They need to know what real information is for their health | |

1.11. ADOLESCENTS' ACCESS TO SEXUAL REPRODUCTIVE HEALTH SERVICES

In the opinion of 9 nurses, adolescents' access to health services in the area of sexual reproductive health is difficult because, according to one nurse

"(...) as these are small communities, when adolescents seek services, even in small numbers, they encounter the barrier of being known by the helper or a neighbor, which leads them to inhibit themselves at all levels" (E7).

Some of them also believe that this difficulty of access is due to the lack of a family nurse at the health center. On the other hand, 40 nurses said that access was very easy and there were no constraints.

From a nurse's perspective:

"The hours are flexible, and the nurses are available and receptive to these issues" (E5).

However, the main issue comes from young people, as most of them feel embarrassed to talk about the subject. Therefore, the majority of nurses believe that schools should also be more active in relation to sexual reproductive health, and even suggest that a nurse should actually be present at the school (see Table 15).

Table 15 - Classification of adolescents' access to health services in the area of sexual reproductive health

Category	Sub-categories	Response indicators	Frequency
Adolescents' access to sexual reproductive health services	Rating out of 1	Very difficult	9
	Rating 4/5	Very easy	40

1.12. THE REAL IMPORTANCE OF NURSES IN RESPONDING TO ADOLESCENTS IN SEXUAL HEALTH

Table 16 shows that all the nurses interviewed (n=49) consider the nurse's role in responding to adolescents' sexual reproductive health to be extremely important, because

"(...) sexuality is present at all ages and nurses have to adapt according to the ages they encounter, the characteristics of each adolescent, considering that each one has their own singularities (.)" (E13).

They are also of the opinion that it is the nurses who have to know how to adapt to the issue.

Table 16 - Nurses' real importance in responding to adolescents' sexual reproductive health

Category	Sub-categories	Response indicators	Frequency
The real importance of nurses in responding to adolescents in sexual reproductive health	A lot of importance	Rating at the top of the scale - 5	49

1.13. HOW THE PROMOTION OF SEXUAL HEALTH IN ADOLESCENCE MAY (OR MAY NOT) CONTRIBUTE TO THE OVERALL WELL-BEING OF ADOLESCENTS NOW AND IN THE FUTURE

Finally, it was found that all the nurses also believe that promoting sexual health in adolescence can clearly contribute to the overall well-being of adolescents now and in the future (see Table 17). According to their unit records,

"(...) the promotion of sexual health in adolescence leads adolescents to know themselves, to gain maturity in relation to the experience of sexuality, making them respect themselves and others, resulting in a more harmonious growth, experiencing their adolescence in a healthier way and a responsible sexuality" (E21).

Also of great importance was the fact that sexual health promotion helps adolescents to value themselves, which will have repercussions in the future. For the nurses,

"(...) sexuality should be seen as a fundamental part of adolescents' lives (...)" (E6).

Promoting sexual health

"(...) it contributes a lot to clarifying friendship, affections, knowing how to distinguish between a dating relationship and, in the future, a relationship between husband and wife" (E10).

Table 17 - How adolescent sexual health promotion can contribute (or not) to the overall well-being of adolescents now and in the future

Category	Sub-categories	Response indicators	Frequency
How adolescent sexual health promotion may (or may not) contribute to the overall well-being of adolescents now and in the future	Contributes to the promotion of present and future well-being	Leads adolescents to get to know themselves Leads adolescents to gain maturity when it comes to experiencing sexuality Makes teenagers respect themselves and others Helps teenagers grow up differently, with responsibility for their actions Helping teenagers to have a healthy adolescence and responsible sexuality Getting teenagers to value themselves	49

1.2 DISCUSSION OF RESULTS

In this subchapter, the most relevant results are discussed, with a critical reflection on them, taking into account the theoretical framework of reference.

From the outset, it should be noted that adolescence is a unique phase of life, associated with childhood experiences and the potential inherent in the adult individual, which characterizes it as a period of significant transformations (Corti & Souza, 2004). This transience, corroborated by the nurses interviewed, is based on the proposition that the majority of adolescents' experiences are linked to preparing them to enter adulthood. However, this idea can be seen as controversial. Even though the transitional nature of adolescence is emphasized in discussions on the subject, the nurses interviewed agreed that adolescence is not limited to future expectations because, after all, adolescents live in their own time, participating in social life and living out their sexuality.

This stage of life sees the acceleration and deceleration of physical growth, changes in body composition, hormonal outbursts, including sex hormones and the development of sexual maturity, accompanied by the development of male and female secondary sexual characteristics. Alongside the bodily changes, psycho-emotional changes arise, such as the search for identity, group tendencies, the development of conceptual thinking, singular experiences and the evolution of sexuality (Oliveira, 2011). The transformations of this phase of life make adolescents live their sexuality intensely, often manifesting it through unprotected sexual practices, which becomes a problem due to a lack of information, communication within the family, taboos or even the fact that they are afraid to assume their sexuality (Pacheco, 2010). The development of their sexual feelings, behaviors and decisions may be influenced by the interactions they develop with other adolescents in their family and social circle, which, in *a way*, neglects the role of nurses.

First of all, according to 29 nurses, the age group that most often seeks health services for sexual issues/problems is the 14-18 age group, 11 nurses mentioned the 15-18 age group and 9 indicated the 18-21 age group. It was also noted that some nurses mentioned another age group, from 10 to 18 years old. However, these adolescents don't go to the health center of their own free will or on the advice of their parents, but because they are summoned for the comprehensive examination, and they go accompanied by their parents. Other nurses also referred to this age group not as adolescents who might go to the health center for sexuality issues, but in a school context, with nurses meeting them more in schools and not the other way around. The results found corroborate the literature, such as the study by Ferreira and Torgal (2011), whose study revealed that few adolescents seek out the Health Center for sexual issues/problems, and that when they do, the predominant age group is 14-18 years old. Bràs (2008), in his study, found that almost all the nurses surveyed said that the age group that most seeks out health services for sexual problems is female adolescents over 15 and under 20, although this varies from health region to health region.

It was found that 34 of the nurses interviewed said that the greatest demand for health services for sexual issues/problems was from girls, which they said could be explained by the fact that they were nurses and boys didn't feel as comfortable, while this was the opposite according to the 4 nurses interviewed, as the demand in their case was predominantly from boys. We also found that 11 of the nurses interviewed said that there was a demand for these services from adolescents of both sexes. This demand is still very low, which in most cases is due to the fact that the Health Centers have adolescents from rural areas as users and also because parents are not receptive to this type of question, with cultural issues and taboos about human sexuality prevailing, which leaves adolescents still very inhibited. It was also argued that the fact that adolescents don't seek out health services is due to the fact that they look for other means of information, such as the internet and their peers.

In this context, and with reference to the study by Bràs (2012), who questioned adolescents about the ideal place to talk to health professionals about problems related to their sexuality, he found that for most girls and boys, the preferred place should be the health center. Comparing this with the results of this study, it can be said that this ideal is not fully realized, since the nurses interviewed agreed that the number of adolescents seeking help is still low. In the study by Bràs (2012), it was shown that most adolescents believe that nurses should be at school, where they spend most of their time, and this was a proposal put forward by one nurse interviewed, according to whom schools should have a permanent nurse on site, as a way of providing adolescents with a space to address questions about their sexuality.

In accordance with the results, and with regard to the reasons that lead adolescents to the Health Center, it was found that all the interviewees said that it is common for adolescents of both sexes to go to the Health Center because of contraceptive methods. Twenty-seven nurses said that the majority of girls also seek information about unwanted pregnancies, while 15 nurses said that adolescents seek information about sexually transmitted infections. Some nurses said that adolescents in the 18-21 age group seek health services, especially girls, because of pregnancy termination and contraceptive issues, while very few boys do so, delegating this responsibility to girls. These results corroborate those of Rodrigues (2014), whose study revealed that, in matters of a sexual nature, the main reasons why adolescents seek out health professionals are contraceptive methods, especially the pill for girls, who are increasingly seeking out the morning-after pill, and for reasons of voluntary termination of pregnancy. This evidence is consistent with the results of the present study, since the search for contraceptive methods was mainly among girls (n=49), followed by voluntary termination of pregnancy, which was considered by 11 nurses to be a borderline situation. Similarly, Brâs (2008) concluded in her study that the overwhelming majority of nurses consider contraception to be the subject most frequently raised by adolescents.

Ferreira and Torgal (2011) point out that it is important for sexually active adolescents to receive health care and advice from health professionals, which requires health institutions and their professionals to be proactive in order to prevent adolescents from engaging in risky behavior, the results of which compromise their development and their current and future health. The authors point out that some risk behaviors result, in particular, in motherhood/paternity, with irreversible consequences. To reinforce this, Bràs, Anes, Praça and Morais (2010), based on their research with 1,735 nurses working in 226 health centers in the 18 health sub-regions of mainland Portugal and the autonomous regions of Madeira and the Azores, found that the majority of nurses (89.9%) usually dealt with adolescents. However, they found that 88.5% had no specific training in sexuality, which led them into risky situations.

In this regard, a significant number of the nurses interviewed believe that adolescents don't talk or seek information about emotional or relational issues. However, the fact that adolescents don't talk about emotional or relational issues with health professionals doesn't mean that they devalue emotions. It has to do, on the one hand, with the representations adolescents have of health services and health professionals, i.e. for many adolescents, doctors and nurses are there to provide contraception, to help with risk situations, but not to talk about "emotional issues", which is usually a subject they discuss with their friends.

The prevailing view was that adolescents don't address affective or relational issues of their own volition, and that this is a topic that is rarely dealt with, and when it is, it's at the urging of nurses, who consider it to be a more complex subject. In this regard, Bràs et al. (2010) point out that sexuality is one of the essential dimensions of the human condition, which is often neglected in educational and health contexts, due to ignorance, cultural prejudices or the supposed defense of individual privacy. As it is one of the most important axes of the human structure, the nurses interviewed admitted that this dimension goes beyond the contingency of relational dynamics to become part of the adolescents' identity through expression and affective involvement. As such, they all reiterate the importance of adolescents knowing about human sexuality in its bio-psycho-social and affective dimensions, having a perfect understanding of their psychosexual and affective development, and understanding the importance of identity formation in the process of sexual differentiation and gender construction, based on respect for themselves and for others. According to them, it is crucial for adolescents to be able to distinguish between the different types of affective bonds during adolescence, as well as to know the signs and impact of situations of violence during adolescence, so that they can lay the foundations for an affective-sexual education that takes their development processes into account.

The registration units of the nurses interviewed clearly showed that affective or relational issues play a fundamental role in human life, as every human being needs physical contact with others, intimacy. It follows that nurses should be attentive to these emotional and affective aspects. For example, an adolescent, regardless of gender, who is visibly upset should be given attention. Situations of violence or exploitation, when reported, should be dealt with and if the nurse doesn't feel prepared, they need to know how to network with other professionals, for example psychologists.

The nurses interviewed admitted that some teenagers have a lot of doubts and a great deal of "inner turmoil", explaining that at this stage of life there are contours that would become more visible if teenagers talked to them about sexuality issues, which they generally don't do, due to inhibition and even social and cultural pressure and because they have information gathered from the Internet and peer groups as a point of reference. One of the specialist nurses argued that "fragility prevails and doubts multiply". They therefore suggest the need to address sexual intimacy with adolescents, emphasizing the difference between three of the affections usually associated with it: sexual desire, attraction and falling in love.

The nurses stressed the importance of adolescents knowing the person they are communicating with sexually, warning them about the danger of immediate relationships. This is a reason for greater investment on the part of health professionals in partnership with the school/parents, since, as emerged from the interviewees' testimonies, this is a topic that is widely discussed in society in general, but little work is done in terms of communication with adolescents in the field.

It was found that 37 nurses rated their comfort/discomfort with each of the sexual topics they discuss with adolescents on a scale of 1 to 5 (where 1 is "Total discomfort" and 5 is "Totally comfortable"), at the maximum point on the scale, justifying this total comfort with the importance of prioritizing these topics with adolescents. However, they point out that it's not an easy task, because many teenagers aren't mature enough and others don't feel open to talking about these issues. For these nurses, sexuality is a topic like any other, with the same importance as any other health issue, and it comes up as naturally as any other topic. It was also found that 12 nurses rated their comfort in talking to adolescents about sexuality at point 4 on the scale, justifying this rating with the fact that adolescents often feel inhibited when they talk about affections, which makes it very difficult or even limits their approach.

As a result, the vast majority of nurses were unanimous in saying that they try to look at adolescents' sexual development from the perspective of their geographical, historical and cultural context. They attach great importance to their role in the approach they give to the sexuality of adolescents, with whom they have daily contact as part of their professional activity, both at the health center and at school. They based their position on the assumption that sexuality and sexual education are two factors that primary health care nurses should take into account. They also justified this with the premise that the health needs of adolescents have very specific characteristics, which are an echo of the process of growth and development with which they are intertwined. The conquest of knowledge, the reorganization of personal identity represent cognitive needs which, alongside affective and sexual motivations, deserve special attention and appreciation, corroborating the opinion of several authors (Marques et al., 2000, Sampaio, 2006; Vaz, 2007).

A large proportion of those interviewed believe that the behavior of many adolescents often involves biological, psychological and social risks. These aspects justify the fact that the actions taken by nurses to promote child and adolescent health should be based on valuing the psychosocial components of biological needs, or vice versa, as Brâs et al. (2010) advocate.

Responding to one of the most frequently asked questions, the nurses interviewed argued that there is no "best age" to start having sex, and even pointed out that the earlier they start having sex, the earlier adolescents are exposed to risks, pointing out that it's not just age that counts, everyone has the right to a different sexual biography, and it's not because colleagues have already had sex that adolescents have to have sex too. These results are in line with those of Bràs (2008), where nurses also considered that there is no fixed age for the start of sexual life. The majority of respondents were of the opinion that the age of first sexual intercourse is getting earlier and earlier, due to social pressure, as stated by the nurses in this study.

At the same time, it was found that the vast majority of information that adolescents obtain is acquired through the internet and their group of friends. The information they do have often has a lot of gaps in it, which adds to adolescents' difficulties when it comes to their own sexuality, in line with what several authors have said (Macpherson, 2001; Sampaio, 2006; Vaz et al., 2007). In this way, the nurses interviewed consider their role in sorting out information to be of crucial importance, as is their approach to affections. In this sense, they argued that sexuality is also linked to affective aspects, life history and cultural values, which contribute to the formation of general identity and to the components of sexual identity, gender identity, gender role and sexual orientation, which are not addressed by the adolescents they come into contact with in their professional practice.

In this context, it is important to note that Caldeira (2008) considers that many adolescents have a lack of knowledge about sexuality, contraceptive methods and sexually transmitted infections, which, according to the author, is associated with a lack of adequate and consistent sexual education. In this respect, the results obtained are also in line with what Soares, Santos and Gonçalves (2011) point out: when adolescents are confronted with a lot of information, which is not always explicit and is sometimes contradictory, they find it difficult to interpret it and in most cases they don't have anyone they can trust to explain it to them properly. In view of this, nurses can take on the role of sexuality educators, helping them to obtain scientific knowledge appropriate to their level of development and equipping them with knowledge that will allow them to choose healthy behaviors when experiencing their sexuality, an opinion corroborated by the vast majority of nurses interviewed.

A person's psychosocial and sexual development, emotional balance and social relationships are all underpinned by their sexual experiences, whether or not they had them during adolescence, a phase in which relationships with family and social groups change, conflicts begin, experimentation starts and, consequently, risky behavior begins. However, it should be noted that our sexuality is not decisively influenced by sexual experiences during adolescence, since our learning is a continuum with advances and setbacks. However, it is essential to remember that sexual experiences during adolescence are important. Family, school and health systems are important links in identifying, supporting and protecting adolescents as they move towards maturity and responsibility for their sexuality (Damas, 2007). In this context, most of the nurses interviewed felt that adolescents should only start their sex lives as long as they feel comfortable with themselves and their partner, as it is a perfectly normal event, an integral part of human development, and one that should be experienced responsibly, pleasurably and on the basis of trust between partners.

The majority of nurses (n=40) said that adolescents' access to health services in the area of sexual reproductive health is very easy and there are no constraints. However, the central issue is that most adolescents feel embarrassed to talk about the subject. As such, they believe that schools should also be more active in relation to sexual reproductive health, with greater intervention on their part.

The results showed that the attitude of nurses towards adolescent sexuality is positive, with nurses (n=49) considering their role in responding to adolescents' sexual reproductive health to be extremely important, as their contribution is crucial to promoting the overall well-being of adolescents now and in the future. In this context, one of the nurses interviewed said that there is no *standard* pedagogy for approaching sexuality in adolescents, emphasizing the idea that all methods/strategies can be valid, as long as they are adapted to each case, and that an example should always be sexuality experienced with the body and all the senses, in a context of reciprocal happiness, affection, care and love, where respect prevails between partners and shared responsibility.

CONCLUSIONS / RECOMMENDATIONS

In this study, we have interwoven some considerations about adolescence, sexuality, sexual education as a task shared by the family, peer group, school and health professionals, as well as the attitude of nurses towards adolescent sexuality.

Promoting sexual and reproductive health involves sex education, which is the specific learning about the elements of adolescent sexuality. This learning takes place as a continuous process throughout the life cycle and includes various components, including physical, psychological, erotic, genital, daily relationships and experimentation, among others. In this sense, the study of nurses' attitudes towards adolescent sexuality made sense. The research question was answered by finding out that the nurses interviewed had a very positive attitude towards adolescent sexuality issues, They were concerned about the fact that the majority of adolescents do not approach affective or relational issues of their own volition, which, according to some interviewees, may be due to the fact that this is a subject that is usually shared with peers and not with health professionals, or because, in the opinion of some interviewees, their relationships are mostly sporadic and temporary rather than effective. It was also concluded that there is a lack of maturity in matters of sexuality on the part of both boys and girls, the effects of the emancipation of women and their greater freedom from society.

The overwhelming majority of nurses said that few adolescents go to the health center for sexual issues, and those who do are motivated by the search for contraceptive methods and unwanted pregnancies. Among the nurses surveyed, it emerged that the age group most likely to seek health services for sexual problems is adolescents over 15 and under 18, especially females. For nurses, contraception is the subject most frequently raised by adolescents. The majority of nurses believe that the beliefs and values conveyed by society influence adolescents' sexual freedom, as well as the sources of information, especially the internet, leading them to seek out nurses more often for contraceptive reasons. The nurses are of the opinion that there should be no age stereotype for the start of sexual life, that it should begin when the adolescent feels ready, despite the need for experimentation typical of the age. They were unanimous in their opinion that most of the time teenagers start their sex lives because of social pressure and because others have already done so at an earlier age.

It was concluded that the overwhelming majority of nurses feel comfortable addressing issues of a sexual nature with adolescents, with the *nuance* that the individual characteristics of each adolescent should always be taken into account, so that interventions can be adapted to their needs. In the same way, most nurses say that promoting sexual health in adolescence contributes to the overall well-being of adolescents now and in the future. However, it is imperative to encourage adolescents that sexuality includes experiences in intimate relationships, which must be lived to the full, with maturity and responsibility.

In view of the results, it is suggested that partnerships between the family, the school and health professionals should be better implemented. This is essential for the success of adolescents who are better informed about sexuality as a whole and, notoriously, more likely to have favorable attitudes towards it. Intervention with more information and greater debate on sexuality are required, as they are aspects that need to be present in the daily lives of adolescents, whether in a school context, a family context or in the context of health services, because only in this way can adolescents have a more favorable attitude towards their sexuality. Nurses' intervention is seen as a tool to help adolescents manage their sexuality in a healthy way.

In view of the results obtained, it is believed that there can be no isolated/punctual educational interventions, which may even be the origin of the way adolescents view their sexuality, devoid of little consistent knowledge, which is why a change in strategies is suggested. In light of the above, it is suggested that a structured intervention project be built in the area of sexuality, based on the directives set out in Law 60/2009 of August 6, regulated by Ministerial Order 196/2010 of April 9, as well as the formation of health support offices in accordance with the law in force, placing greater emphasis on the importance of making adolescents responsible for their sexuality. It is also important to implement dynamic strategies and interventions in health centers to encourage adolescents to seek health services about sexuality issues, especially in relation to affections.

Finally, as well as being a great contribution to personal growth, this work is also a professional asset, serving as support for restructuring intervention projects in the community, as a time to review strategies and plan new interventions. It is suggested that further research be carried out in this area, which could give continuity to the study of nurses' attitudes towards sexuality in adolescents, fostering a healthy sexual experience, not only physically but also psychologically, and therefore promoting individual and collective health.

BIBLIOGRAPHY

Albuquerque, C. (2004). *Health and Risk Behavior in Adolescence: Psychosocial and Cognitive Determinants.* PhD thesis. Spain: University of Extremadura.

Alferes, V.R. (1997). *Staging and Sexual Behavior.* Porto: Ediçoes Afrontamento.

Alves, C. A. (2010). *The Impact of a Sex Education Program on Adolescents' Protective Behaviors.* Available at: http://repositorio-aberto.up.pt/bitstream/10216/55445/2/TeseCristianaAlves.pdf

Antunes, M. (2007). *Sexual attitudes and behaviors of higher education students.* Coimbra: Formasau.

Avery, L., & Lazdane, G. (2008). What do we know about sexual and reproductive health of adolescents in Europe? *The European Journal of Contraception & Reproductive Health Care,* Ternat, v. 13, 1: 58-70.

Bardin, L. (2004). *Content Analysis.* Lisbon: ediçoes 70.

Belo, M.A.V., & Silva, J.L.P. (2004). Knowledge, attitude and practice about contraceptive methods among pregnant adolescents. *Revista Brasileira de Saùde Pùblica, 38*: 479487.

Berger, K.S. (2003). *The development of the person from childhood to adolescence.* 5. ed. Rio de Janeiro: LTC.

Bobak, I., Lowdermilk, D. & Jensen, M. (2007). *Maternity Nursing.* 6ª ed.

Lisbon: Lusociência.

Bogdan, R. & Biklen, S. (1994). *Investigaçao qualitativa em* educaçao - Colecçao ciências da educaçao, Porto: Porto Editora.

Braconnier, A., & Marcelli, D. (2007). *The thousand faces of adolescence.* Lisbon. Climepsi Editores.

Bràs, M. F. M. (2012). *Sexuality in Adolescence: analysis of the adolescent's perspective on sexuality.* Accessed at: https://bibliotecadigital.ipb.pt/handle/10198/8008

Bràs, M.A.M (2008). *Adolescent Sexuality: The perspective of Primary Health Care Nursing Professionals.* PhD Thesis in Nursing Sciences, University of Porto. ICBAS. Porto.

Bràs, M.A.M., Anes, E.M.G.J., Praça, M.I.F. & Morais, M.F. (2010). Adolescents and sexuality: issues in the search for primary health care. *International Journal of Developmental and Educational Psychology INFAD. Revista de Psicologia,* Vol.2 1: 413-422

Bràs. M. & Azevedo, Z. (2009). *The Perspective of Primary Health Care Nursing Professionals on Adolescent Sexuality: Development and validation of a scale.* Accessed March, 09, 2013: available at https://bibliotecadigital.ipb.pt/bitstream/10198/3547/1/Artigo-Manuel_Bràs.pdf

Caldeira, E.C. (2008). Sexual behaviors of adolescents. *Servir,* Vol. 53, 1: 29-39.

Canavarro, M.C., & Pereira, A.I. (2001). Pregnancy and motherhood in adolescence: theoretical perspectives. In M. C. Canavarro (Ed.), *Psicologia da gravidez e da maternidade* (pp. 323-355). Coimbra: Quarteto Editora.

Cardoso, S., Rodrigues, A. Nelas, P., & Duarte, J. (2010). Educating for responsible sexuality in adolescence. *Journal of the Portuguese Association of Obstetric Nurses,* 11, 9-14.

Carvalho, A. M., Rodrigues, C. S., & Medrado, K. S. (2005). Workshops on human sexuality with adolescents. *Estudos de Psicologia*, 10(3): 377-384.

Cervo, A. and Bervian, P. (1983). *Metodologia Científica* (3ª ed.). Sao Paulo: McGraw-Hill.

Correia, F.T.A. (2013). *Adolescents and sexuality: knowledge and attitudes*. Master's dissertation. Escola Superior de Saùde de Viseu. Acedido em:http://repositorio.ipv.pt/bitstream/10400.19/1991/1/CORREIA,%20Toni%20Fernando%20 Aguilar%20%20disserta%C3%A7%C3%A3o%20mestrado%20EMBARGO%2019%20junho% 202014.pdf

Costa, A.J.L.L. da (2006). *Sexual education from a health education perspective: an exploratory study at the Santa Maria Maior Secondary School in Viana do Castelo*. Master's dissertation. University of Minho. Institute of Education and Psychology. Accessed on:

https://repositorium.sdum.uminho.pt/bitstream/1822/6284/3/DISSERTA%C3%87%C3%83O% 20de%20Mestrado.pdf

Costa, S.F.P. (2015). *Knowledge, attitudes and beliefs regarding sexuality and sexual education of 8th and 10th grade adolescents*. Master's dissertation. Nursing School of Porto   . Accessed at: http://comum.rcaap.pt/bitstream/10400.26/10779/1/Tese%20Sandra%20Costa%20.pdf.

Cuesta Benjumea, C. de la (2001). Contexto del embarazo en la adolescencia: nos hicimos novios y ahi empezó todo. *Revista Rol de Enfermeria*. Barcelona. Vol. 24, 9: 24-30.

Damas, M. (2007). *Good Practice Guide. Adoles (Being). Sexuality and Affections*. Accessed at: http://www.dge.mec.pt/sites/default/files/Esaude/guia_adoles_ser.pdf

Decree-Law no. 259/2000, of October 17th. Official Gazette no. 240 - Series I-A

Dias, S. (2013). *Sexual Education in schools in the municipality of Oeiras: Perception of teachers and students*. Lisbon: Technical University of Lisbon - Faculty of Human Motricity.

Directorate-General for Health (2013). National Child and Youth Health Program. Accessed at: http://www.dgs.pt/documentos-e-publicacoes/programa-tipo-de-atuacao-em-saude-infantil-e- juvenil.aspx

Ferreira, M.M.S.R.S. & Torgal, M.C.L.F.P.R. (2011). Lifestyles in adolescence: sexual behavior of Portuguese adolescents. *Rev Esc Enferm USP*, 45(3): 589-95.

Flick, U. (2005). *Qualitative Methods in Scientific Research*. 2.ª ed.. Lisbon: Monitor.

Flora, M. C., Rodrigues, R. F. F. & Paiva, H. M. C. G. da C. (2013). Sexual education interventions for adolescents: a systematic literature review. *Revista de Enfermagem Referência, ser III* (10): 125-134.

Fonseca, E.B.M., & Machado, A.J.B.B. (2007). Affective/emotional skills in adolescents' experience of sexuality. *Vital Signs*. Coimbra, 72: 25-27, ISSN 0872-8844.

Fonseca, H. (2005). *Understanding Adolescents - A challenge for parents and educators*. 4ª edition. Barcarena: Editorial Presença.

Fonseca, H. (2010). *Living with teenagers*. Lisbon: Editorial Presença.

Fonseca, L., Soares, C. & Vaz, J. (2003). *A Sexologia Perspetiva Multidisciplinar II* (Vol 1, pp.117 - 155). Coimbra: Quarteto Editora.

Fortin, M.F. (2009). *Fundamentals and stages of the research process*. Loures: Lusodidata.

Freixo, M.J.V. (2011). *Metodologia Científica - Fundamentos Métodos e Técnicas*. 3ª Edition. Lisbon: Instituto Piaget.

Gouveia, Patricia et al. (2010). Scale of motivation to have and not to have sex: adolescent version. In Leal, Isabel; Maroco, Joao. *Assessment in sexuality and parenting*. Lisbon: Livpsic.

Sexual Education Working Group (2007). *Final report*. Accessed at: www.dgidc.min-edu.pt/educacaosaude/.../educacaosaude/educacaosexual.

Hockenberry, M.W.D., Wilson, & Winklestein, M. (2014). *Wong fundamentals of pediatric nursing*. Elsevier: Rio de Janeiro.

Johnson, D. (1999). *Body*. Rio de Janeiro: Nova Fronteira.

Kaplan, H., Sadock, B., & Grebb, J. (2007). *Compendium of Psychiatry: Behavioral Science and Clinical Psychiatry* (9th ed.). Porto Alegre: Artes Médicas.

Kirby, J., Van der Sluijs, W., & Currie, C. (2010). *HBSC Briefing Supplement 18b: Attitudes towards condom use among young people. Child and Adolescent Health Research* Unit. The University of Edinburgh. HBSC Briefing Paper Series.

Lakatos, E. V. & Marconi, M. A. (2004). *Metodologia científica.* Sao Paulo: Editora Atlas.

Law no. 60/2009. D.R. I Series. 151 (2009-8-6) 5097-5098. Establishes the system for applying sex education in schools.

LoBiondo - Wood, G. & Haber, J. (2001). *Nursing Research - Methods, Evaluation, Criticism and Utilization* (4ª ed.). Rio de Janeiro: Editora Guanabara Koogan.

López, F. S. & Fuertes, A. M. (1997). *Aproximaciones Al Estudio de La Sexualidad* (1ª ed). Salamanca: Amarù Ediciones.

López, F. S. (2005). *Sexual education*. Madrid: Editorial Biblioteca Nueva.

López, F.S. & Fuertes, A.M. (1999). *Understanding sexuality*. Lisbon: Family Planning Association.

Marques, A. C. (2009). *Men are not equal and all women are not equal: young people's representations of sexuality*. Accessed at

http://repositorio.iscte.pt/bitstream/10071/1537/1/CIESWP76%20Marques.pdf

Martins, A.T., Nunes, C., Munoz-Silva, A., & Sànchez-Garcia, M. 2008. Sources of information, knowledge and condom use in university students from Algarve and Huelva. *Psico* 39:7-13.

Martins, M.M.B.P. (2010). *Knowledge and behavior about some sexually transmitted infections among primary and secondary school students in a school in the greater Lisbon area*. Master's dissertation. New University of Lisbon. Institute of Hygiene and Tropical Medicine. Accessed at: http://run.unl.pt/bitstream/10362/13997/1/v-final%206.6.pdf

Matos, M. G., Simoes, C., Vilar, D. et al. (2010). *Sexualidade Afectos e Cultura - Gestão de problemas de saúde em meio escolar* (1ª ed.). Lisbon: Coisas de Ler.

Matos, M.G., Reis, M., Ramiro, L., & Equipa Aventura Social (2012). *Sexual and Reproductive Health of Higher Education Students, Study Report - National Data 2010*. Lisbon: National Coordination for HIV/AIDS Infection/High Commissioner for Health - Ministry of Education; CMDTla/IHMT/UNL; FMH/UTL; FCT/MCTES; IPJ; Portal Sapo. Accessed at: www.aventurasocial.com.

Matos, M.G., Sampaio, D., Baptista, I. & Equipa Aventura Social, UTL and CMDT/UNL (2013). Adolescent's health education and promotion in Portugal: a case study of planning for sustainable practice. In Samdal, O., & Rowling, L. (Eds.), *The Implementation of health promoting schools, exploring theories of what, why and how* (pp.123-126). New York: Routledge Taylor & Francis Group.

Mota, C. P. (2008). *Relational dimensions in the psychosocial adaptation process of adolescents: Vulnerability and resilience in institutionalization, divorce and intact families*. PhD thesis. Faculty of Psychology and Educational Sciences, University of Porto, Porto.

Nelas, P. (2011). Sexual education in schools: the impact of participatory and reflective methodologies. *European Journal of Public Health*.Volume 21. Supplement 1, p.71.

Nelas, P., Fernandes, C., Ferreira, M., Duarte, J. & Chaves, C. (2011).*Knowledge of adolescents about contraceptive methods: Impact of one training intervention. International Conference on Education & Educational Psychology*. Abstracts Book, Vol. 2, [Abstract].

Nelas, P., Fernandes, C., Ferreira, M., Duarte, J. & Chaves, C. (2010). *Construction and validation of the scale of attitudes towards sexuality in adolescents (AFSA). Sexuality and sex education: educational policies, research and practices* (1ª ed.). Accessed at http://www.fpccsida.org.pt/images/stories/Livro_I_CISES.pdf

Nelas, P.A.A.B. (2010). *Sexual Education in the School Context*. PhD thesis. University of Aveiro. Department of Educational Sciences. Accessed at: https://core.ac.uk/download/files/580/15564830.pdf

Neto, F. (1998). *Psicologia Social* (Vol.1, pp. 337). Lisbon: Universidade Aberta.

Nodin, N. (2001). Portuguese youth and sexuality at the end of the 20th century. Lisbon, Portugal: APF. Polit, D. F; Hungler, B. P. *Fundamentals of nursing research* (3ª ed). Porto Alegre, Brazil: Artes Médicas.

Oliveira, V.C.M. (2011). *Adolescent Sexuality - Motivation for having or not having sex*. Master's dissertation. Escola Superior de Saúde de Viseu. Accessed at:

http://repositorio.ipv.pt/bitstream/10400.19/1572/1/OLIVEIRA%20Vera%20Cristina%20Madei ra,%20Sexualidade%20adolescente.pdf.

Oliveira, V.C.M. de, Nelas, P., Aparicio, G. & Duarte, J. (2014). Adolescents' sexual motivation: influence of sociodemographic factors. *Millenium*, 46: 197-210. Accessed at: http://www.ipv.pt/millenium/Millenium46/12.pdf

Ordem dos Enfermeiros (2010). *Sexuality, Adolescence and Health.* Accessed at: http://www.ordemenfermeiros.pt/sites/acores/artigospublicadoimpressalocal/Paginas/%E2%80 %9CSEXUALITY,ADOLESC%C3%8ANCIAESA%C3%9ADE.aspx.

Ordem dos Enfermeiros (2015) *Statistical Yearbook 2014.* Accessed at: http://www.ordemenfermeiros.pt/Documents/DadosEstatisticos/Estatistica_V01_2014.pdf

Pacheco, P., Mota, I. & Clemente, P. (2010). *Sexuality, adolescence and health.* Azores: Ordem dos Enfermeiros. Accessed at http://www.ordemenfermeiros.pt/sites/acores/artigospublicadoimpressalocal/Paginas/"SEXUALITY,ADOL ESCENCEANDHEALTH.aspx

Paixao, P. (2005). The bê-a-ba of sex in adolescence. *Sàbado Revista*, 37: 36-47.

Polit, D.F. & Hungler, B.P. (2004). *Fundamentals of nursing research* (3ª ed.). Porto Alegre: Artes Médicas.

Pontes, A.F. (2011). *Sexuality: let's talk about it? Promoting Psychosexual Development in Adolescence: Implementation and Evaluation of a School-based Intervention Program.* Master's dissertation. Abel Salazar Institute of Biomedical Sciences, University of Porto. Accessed at: https://repositorio-aberto.up.pt/bitstream/10216/24432/2/Sexualidade%20vamos%20conversar%20sobre%20isso.p df.

Portaria n.° 196-A/2010, de 9 de abril- Diàrio da Repûblica, 1.ª série - N.° 69 - 9 de Abril de 2010.

Prazeres, V., Laranjeira, A., Marques, A. et al. (2005). *National Youth Health Program 2006/2010. Lisbon: Directorate-General for Health, Maternal, Child and Adolescent Health Division.* Accessed on April 05, 2013 at Direção Geral da Saúde: Available at http://www.ordemenfermeiros.pt/sites/acores/artigospublicadoimpressalocal/Paginas/"SEXUAL AGE,ADOLESCENCE AND HEALTH.aspx

Ramiro, L.I.S. da (2013). *Sexual education in changing adolescents' sexual knowledge, attitudes and behaviors.* PhD thesis. Technical University of Lisbon. Faculty of Human Motricity. Accessed at: https://www.repository.utl.pt/bitstream/10400.5/5862/1/Lucia_Ramiro_Dout.pdf

Ramos, A. L. (2003). *Citizen empowerment in health: what is the role of the health professional? What is the citizen's perception?* National School of Public Health, University of Lisbon. Lisbon: Repository of the New University of Lisbon. Master's dissertation.

Ramos, Rui Deveza et al. (2008). *Attitudes, communication and behavior towards sexuality in a population of young people from Matosinhos.* Archives of Medicine. Lisbon. ISSN 0871-3413. Vol. 22, n° 1.

Reis, M. & Matos, M.G. (2008). Sexual behaviours and the influence of different socialization agents on the sexual education of young university students. *Sexuality and Planning*

Familiar, 48/49, 22-28. Available at:

http://aventurasocial.com/arquivo/1303596808_SPFAM_REIS_2008.pdf

Richardson, R. J. (1989). *Social Research: Methods and Techniques* (2ª ed.). Sao Paulo: Atlas.

Rodrigues, C. (2014). *Health education with 3rd grade students and parent-child mediation in a secondary school.* Master's dissertation. University of Minho. Accessed at: http://repositorium.sdum.uminho.pt/bitstream/1822/34893/1/Relat%C3%B3rio%20de%20est%C3%A1gio-%20C%C3%ADntia%20Rodrigues.pdf

Roque, O. (2010). *Semiotics of the stork. Young people, sexuality and the risk of unwanted pregnancy.* Lisbon: Family Planning Association.

Sà, E. (2007). What would become of the sex of Angels if there were Parabolics in Heaven? Lisbon: Press Mundo.

Sampaio, D. (2006). *Lavrar o Mar* (1.ª ed). Lisbon: Editorial Caminho.

Sampaio, D. (2011). *Family, school and a few other things.* Lisbon: Editorial Caminho.

Sampaio, D., Baptista, M., Matos, M. & Silva, M. (2007). *Final Report. Sexual Education Working Group.* Lisbon: Ministry of Education. Directorate-General for Innovation and Curriculum Development.

Sampaio, F. M., & Silva, D. B. (2006). *Sexuality of Portuguese adolescents from the perspective of the "Quebrese: Brief questionnaire on sexuality".* In Proceedings of the XI International Conference, Psychological Assessment, Forms and Contexts. Braga: Psiquilibrios.

Sampieri, R.H., Collado, C.F., Lucio, P.B. & Pérez, M. de la C. (2006). *Metodologia de la investigación.* La Habana: Ciencias Médicas.

Silva, A. (2004). *Development of Social Skills in Adolescents.* Lisbon: Climepsi Editores.

Silva, A.S. & Deus, A.A. (2005). Hashish consumption behaviors and mental health in adolescents: A comparative study. *Anàlise Psicològica, 23*(2): 151-172.

Soares, F.M.F.S., Santos, M.F. & Gonçalves, J.H.G. (2011). *I International Congress on Sexuality and Sex Education. Education for sexuality.* Sexual Education Office (Intervention   Intervention-Action Project). Accessed at: repositorio.esenfc.pt/private/index.php?process=download&id..

Sousa, B.L., & Ferreira, S. J. (2003) - Adolescents' Attitude towards Sexuality. *Revista Sinais Vitais.* Vol. 48: 35-38.

Sousa, M.F.G. (2000). *Sexuality in adolescence.* Master's dissertation. University of Porto. Abel Salazar Institute of Biomedical Sciences. Accessed at: https://bibliotecadigital.ipb.pt/.../Sexualidade%20na%20Adolescência.pdf

Sprinthall, N. A., & Collins, W. A. (2008).*Psicologia do Adolescente*. Lisbon: Calouste Gulbenkian Foundation.

Sprinthall, N. A., & Collins, W. A. (2008).*Psicologia do Adolescente*. Lisbon: Calouste Gulbenkian Foundation.

Stroebe, W. & Hewstone, M. (2001). *Introduction to Social Psychology* (3°ed.).Berlin: Blackwell Publishing.

Tomey, A. M. & Alligood, M. R. (2011). *Models and theories in nursing* (7 ed.). Barcelona: Elsevier Mosby.

Vaz, J. M. (2007). *Eyes to eyes. Stories of sex and life.* Buenos Aires. Boocket Publishing.

Vesley, S.K., Wayatt, V.H., Oman, R.F., Aspy, C.B., Kegler, M.C., Rodine, S., Marshall, L. & Mcleary, K.R. (2004). The potential protective effects of youth assets from adolescent sexual risk behaviors. *Journal of Adolescent Health*, 34: 356-365.

Vieira, O.C.F. (2009). *A Educação Sexual na Escola Pùblica Portuguesa: Um olhar a partir da experiência de alunos do 10° ano*. Master's dissertation. University of Minho. Institute of Education and Psychology. Accessed at: https://repositorium.sdum.uminho.pt/bitstream/1822/11138/1/Tese.pdf.

Vieira, R.V. (2015). *Sexuality in Adolescence: Implementation of a Guidance Program for Students with Intellectual Disabilities*. Master's dissertation. Fernando Pessoa University. Accessed on:

http://bdigital.ufp.pt/bitstream/10284/4770/1/1.%20TESE%20RITA%20VIEIRA.pdf

Vilar, D (2005). Educaçao Sexual em Rede (N°1, July/September, rev.). Lisbon: APF.

Vilar, D. & Ferreira, P. (2009). The sexual education of young Portuguese people: knowledge and sources. *Revista Educaçao Sexual em Rede*, 5, 2-53. Accessed at: http://www.apf.pt/?area=002&mid=004&sid=004

Vilar, D. & Ferreira, P.M. (2009). The sexual education of young Portuguese: Knowledge and sources. *Educaçao Sexual em Rede*, 5: 2-53. Accessed at:

http://www.apf.pt/cms/files/conteudos/file/Anexos%20EDS/Educacao%20Sexual%20em%20R ede/Educacao%20Sexual%20em%20Rede%20AprilSeptember%202009.zip

Vilar, D. & Souto, E. (2008). *Sexual Education in the Context of Professional Training. Referenciais de Formaçao Pedagógica Continua de Formadores/as.* Accessed at: http://opac.iefp.pt:8080/images/winlibimg.exe?key=&doc=45440&img=260

Vilar, D. (2003). *Talking About It, Sex Education in Adolescents' Families*. Porto. Collection: Biblioteca das Ciências do Homem/Sociologia e Epistemologia/38, Afrontamento.

APPENDICES

DECLARATION OF INFORMED CONSENT TO PARTICIPATE IN THE STUDY

Me,

I hereby declare that I have been properly informed about the nature, procedures and form of development of the study on "Nurses' attitudes towards adolescent sexuality", developed within the scope of the Master's Degree in Child Health and Pediatrics being held at the Escola Superior de Saùde da Guarda, Instituto Politècnico da Guarda, and that I understand its contribution to the field.

I was also informed of the guarantee of confidentiality and anonymity of all data.

I further declare that participation in the study is voluntary and I am guaranteed the possibility of refusing to take part at any time, without any justification or consequences.

I hereby declare my free and informed consent to take part in this study, allowing the data I voluntarily provide to be used, trusting that it will only be used for the purpose of the research and the guarantees of confidentiality and anonymity given to me by the researcher.

Date:__/__/__

Signature: _______________

INTERVIEW GUIDE FOR NURSES

1. Individual characterization

Age **48**

Sex **F**

Academic qualifications: **nurse with a specialty in community health**

Length of service **21 years**

Length of service at the current Health Center **21**

Professional category **Nurse**

2. Nurses' attitudes towards adolescent sexuality

1. Which age groups most often seek health services for sexual issues/problems?

2. Which gender adolescents come to the health center most often? Why do they come?

3. Are the reasons why adolescents go to the health center the same for both sexes? If not, what are

the differences?

4. Which risk situations in terms of adolescent SRH appear most frequently in adolescent care?

5. What sexual content is most often covered by teenagers?

6. In relation to each of the subjects you mentioned, and on a scale of 1 to 5 (where 1 is "Total discomfort" and 5 is "Totally comfortable"), how would you rate your comfort/discomfort in dealing with them? Why?

7. In general, what do you think about sexual relationships between teenagers?

8. In your opinion, is there an age at which you should start having sex?

9. How do issues of sexual orientation (homosexual, heterosexual, bisexual, transsexual) come up in adolescent care? How do you usually deal with them?

10. In your approach to sexual issues with adolescents, do you also address issues related to adolescents' affections, feelings and emotional relationships? What kind of issues arise? Are they different between boys and girls? How do you address them?

11. How do you rate the level of knowledge and information that adolescents have about issues related to sexuality? Are there different levels of information and knowledge among young people? Are there differences between boys and girls? What other differences can you identify?

12. On a scale of 1 to 5 (where 1 means very difficult and 5 means very easy), how would you rate adolescents' access to health services in the area of SRH? Please justify.

13. On a scale of 1 to 5, how important are nurses in responding to adolescents with SRH? Justify.

14. How can promoting sexual health in adolescence contribute (or not) to the overall well-being of adolescents now and in the future?

Authorizations for data collection

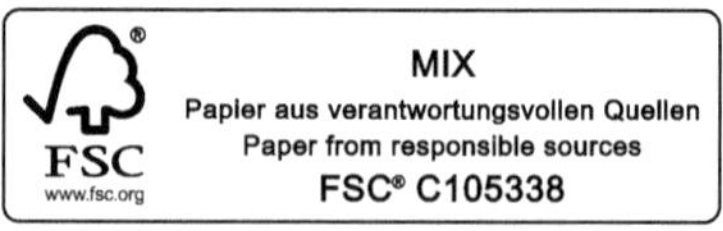

Printed by Books on Demand GmbH, Norderstedt / Germany